YOU'VE GOT THIS

A Student's Guide to Well-being at University and Beyond

To order, or for details of our bulk discounts, please go to our website www.criticalpublishing.com or contact our distributor, Ingram Publisher Services (IPS UK), 10 Thornbury Road, Plymouth PL6 7PP, telephone 01752 202301 or email IPSUK.orders@ingramcontent.com.

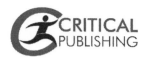

YOU'VE GOT THIS

A Student's Guide to Well-being at University and Beyond

RACHAEL ALEXANDER

British Library Cataloguing in Publication Data
A CIP record for this book is available from the British Library

ISBN: 9781914171260

This book is also available in the following e-book formats:

EPUB ISBN: 9781914171277
Adobe e-book ISBN: 9781914171284

Cover and text design by Fiachra McCarthy
Project Management by Deanta Global Publishing Services, Dublin, Ireland
Typeset by Deanta Global Publishing Services, Chennai, India
Printed and bound in Great Britain by 4edge, Essex

Critical Publishing
3 Connaught Road
St Albans
AL3 5RX

www.criticalpublishing.com

Printed on FSC accredited paper

CONTENTS

WHAT DO I NEED HELP WITH?

ACKNOWLEDGEMENTS

You've Got This manifested into physical form through the power of belief. Thank you to David Gray (UKAT – UK Advising and Tutoring) who, after believing in my ideas, introduced me to Julia Morris at Critical Publishing. Thank you to Julia and team who, after reading my proposal, believed in my voice adding value and supported me in the writing of the book. And, finally, thank you to my earthbound and spiritual soul family who wouldn't let me stop believing in myself. May you, dear reader, like me, always believe in yourself and know you are always fully supported by the divine intelligence which surrounds you, even though at times it may not appear so. And finally, always remember you've got this!

ABOUT THE AUTHOR

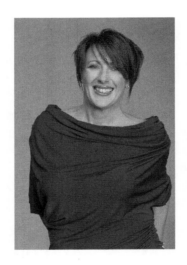

Rachael has qualifications in counselling psychology, cognitive behavioural therapy and consciousness psychology. During her 20-year career working with the NHS, industry, retail, education and mental health charities she has helped thousands to live their lives with resilience, integrity and love. Sharing her own challenges, experiences and acquired wisdom, Rachael demonstrates how self-development and spiritual awareness are the keys to courageously transforming your life to one of action, confidence, faith and trust.

FOREWORD

As someone who grew up in a very dysfunctional household and who struggled through his school years and young adult life, this book resonated with me. Helping young people who are struggling and looking for direction is something close to my heart.

It is an excellent guide to help students through a potentially difficult and challenging time in their lives. If I had been given some of the guidance and help this book offers at that age, my life would've been very different. I fell through a hole and was kicked out of school with no qualifications and very few prospects in life. Drink and drugs became a sanctuary for me and I sank into a very low vibrational place. I also struggled with a lack of self-esteem and made many bad decisions.

Rachael's advice and guidance are also infused with spiritual wisdom and knowledge from her own journey overcoming difficulty to create a successful life. You learn a lot on this kind of journey, and it is a common theme among therapists who are successful in their careers. There is no substitute for having been a fully paid-up student at the open university of real life. Failure and hardship can be great teachers.

This book will help you navigate through many of the pitfalls that young people typically face at a formative age. Having an awareness of the potential we have as human beings can change the course of your life. With this kind of knowledge, you can take full control of your health and mental well-being and avoid the cycle of dependency and reliance on the system that many fall into.

Looking after your own health and well-being is key to living a happy and abundant life. With the right guidance, you can live a self-empowered life where you are in control of your own destiny. You can experience higher realms of consciousness when you work on your inner self and cultivate self-discipline. This is the way to live a truly empowered and ultimately enlightened life.

I went from a life of struggle, low self-esteem, financial hardship and addiction into a life of health, success and abundance. Anyone can do the same with the right guidance, and Rachael's book points you in the direction of self-empowerment, independence and self-love. It has everything you need to navigate the challenges of life, but more than that it will show you how to thrive and prosper and live a truly abundant and happy life.

Young people have so much potential, but often this remains untapped because of self-doubt or conditioned patterns of behaviour that are unresolved. Knowing you can break free from these can be so liberating. Releasing trauma and negative conditioning allows you to grow and live freely without being bogged down by baggage from the past. When you are free in this way, life becomes easier and opportunities manifest everywhere. When your vibrational energy is high you naturally attract people and situations that match that frequency.

Knowing and understanding that you're a powerful human being with infinite potential is life changing. When you create this feeling and learn how to control your mind and ego-self, you begin to set yourself free. The healing journey starts now with this book; I thoroughly recommend it.

Remember to let go of old wounds and traumas or any sabotage patterns; be aware of your shadow self and make wise choices and decisions that align you with things of a high vibrational nature. Live your life to the full and go beyond fear and self-doubt. Be kind and loving to others but also stand your ground and be strong and courageous when you need to be. Speak your truth always. As John Lennon once said, *'telling the truth will not get you a lot of friends but it will get you the right ones'*.

One of the biggest regrets people have at the end of their lives is not taking enough chances and not loving enough; remember that always. Live life from your heart as much as you can, be kind and compassionate and remember that every good deed you do has a ripple effect with an impact on others. Think of the karmic imprint you want to create in the world. Life is a gift and full of opportunities. Make wise choices every step of the way and life will flow!

Good luck and I hope you get everything you need from this book.

Glenn Harrold
Author and hypnotherapist

INTRODUCTION

You've always had the power my dear — you just had to learn it for yourself.

Glenda the Good Witch (Wizard of Oz)

WHY HAS *YOU'VE GOT THIS* BEEN WRITTEN?

After spending many years coaching clients, I understand how difficult it is for a person to take charge of changing a situation, no matter how much emotional pain it is causing. One of the reasons we are resistant to change is fear. Examples of fears stopping people from changing situations include fear of upsetting others, of not being liked, conflict, confrontation, disapproval, feeling a failure and fear of being judged by others. Fear can literally stop you in your tracks.

It is common to suffer experiences as a child which make you feel scared. If you are not taught how to process this fear, you grow up with a fear of fear, thereby living in a constant state of agitation and experiencing emotional pain. This means that then as an adult when faced with challenging situations, and because of your subconscious fears, you might doubt your ability to handle the consequences of taking action and therefore stay stuck, meaning your mental health slowly deteriorates.

For many years I was the same as my clients — scared of facing difficult situations and therefore stayed in emotional pain. I became so used to living this way that my only relief would be to drink alcohol to numb the painful feelings. But, of course, alcohol only offered me temporary relief from this pain. I didn't know it at the time, but I had many fears leading to a huge lack of confidence, and I didn't trust my ability to deal with overwhelming situations.

Attending university can be a worrying time for many students and so is an ideal time for you to learn how to deal courageously with different situations. This then allows you to experience great mental health and well-being, not only while at university but for the rest of your life. I hope that *You've Got This* will help you realise you are not damaged or broken or need fixing in any way simply because you might suffer with uncomfortable feelings, stress or anxiety. If you can learn to think, feel and behave in empowering ways, you can and will become more calm, peaceful and untroubled.

HOW CAN THIS BOOK HELP YOU?

I suggest psychological and spiritual ways to deal with many different life situations you are likely to encounter while at university. Spiritual, as I define it, does not mean religious; it is about knowing you are more than just a human body, but a soul who is here to learn many great lessons, not least about loving yourself and others. Interchangeably I use the terms *Higher Power*, *Universe* or *Divine intelligence*. Yet if you believe in a loving God then please use the language which resonates with you. Some of my clients prefer to use *The Force*, as in Star Wars, or even Spirit Guides. Just think about words with which you are comfortable.

I also use the words *anxiety* and *fear* interchangeably. After years of research and from my own personal experience, these two words mean the same thing to me. For example, if I say, '*I have social anxiety which means I can't mix with people*', I then avoid mixing with people, thinking I have a *disorder* of some kind. With this mindset, I can think anxiety is more powerful than me and that I am damaged or flawed in some way. Granted the physiological symptoms are very real and scary but they should not have the power to control choices and dictate my actions.

However, if I reframe the original statement into '*I am fearful, and my fear makes it hard for me to mix with people*', this simple change of language makes it a much more empowering statement. This is because I can learn to face my fears by moving out of my comfort zone and practise mixing with people. The more I do this, the easier it becomes, and the anxiety/fear disappears. Simply changing the language we use can be incredibly helpful.

INTRODUCTION

HOW THIS BOOK WORKS

....

The book is divided into ten chapters offering structured questions and answers which share simple and practical ways to deal with experiences you may encounter at university. You do not need to start at the beginning of the book, but simply find a situation you are struggling with and read the suggested topic. At the end of each topic are five journal prompts to help you process what you have read and apply it to your own experience. Feel free to scribble your answers in the book, or you may like to write them in a special notebook or type them up. It doesn't matter where you write your answers as long as you do. This is an effective way to reach clarity and a practice which has helped me throughout my life.

There are no wrong answers to these questions; it is simply a process to help you discover more about the way you think, feel and behave and allow you to gain clarity on what your next steps could be. This self-knowledge encourages you to be honest with yourself about what you are thinking and feeling instead of avoiding making decisions, helping to reduce the mental and emotional turmoil you may feel.

You might like to highlight any sentences in the book which are particularly relevant to you to help reinforce your learning. There is also an affirmation in each journal section – repeat this to yourself regularly to help reframe your negative thoughts into positive ones. The journal section ends with a life lesson because the psychological maturity you are developing at university is transferable to other situations in your life.

DO NOT SUFFER IN SILENCE

....

In many of the answers, you will see I am a big advocate of reaching out for help. Over the years I have been very lucky to have the support of many kind and wise souls; mentors, teachers, friends, bosses, colleagues, counsellors, coaches, astrologers, psychics, mediums and a whole myriad of energy healers. There have been times in my life when I have not wanted to continue my human journey, but different people at different stages in my life have psychologically picked me up, dusted me off and sent me back out on my way, emotionally bruised but reignited. I am so thankful to these people and encourage you to find people in whom you can confide.

THE BENEFITS OF TALKING AND TABLETS

I also want to be upfront about my views regarding the use of psychiatric medication such as anti-depressants and anti-anxiety tablets. While some tablets may help some people feel better, it is my personal belief that it is valuable to take the time to explore the way you think and feel. Supporting my belief are guidelines issued for consultation (November 2021) by the National Institute for Health Care and Excellence (NICE). They state that patients should first be offered group classes in things such as meditation, behavioural therapy or individual counselling sessions and should not be routinely offered anti-depressant medication as a first-line treatment for less severe depression unless that is the person's preference.

Talking to a doctor is often the first step in accessing help and you can work together to help you make an informed decision by considering all the different treatment options available. Aim for informed consent which is an interactive agreement between yourself and your doctor on the most suitable course of treatment for you, so that you understand the risks and benefits of taking medication. There are resources in the further reading section of this book which can also help you understand why informed consent is so important.

Of course, as a spiritual psychologist I recommend you also consider alternative ways to help heal yourself and some of these ways are listed throughout the book and in the resources section. While you may not have encountered some of these methods before, they have helped me stay alcohol and medication free while traversing some extremely difficult and traumatic times. However, the most important thing to remember is that it takes courage to reach out for help and you have a right to make the right decision about the best treatment option for you.

From one brave warrior to another, I thank you for taking the time to read *You've Got This* and trust it helps you realise, whatever happens, you've got this.

Rachael Alexander
rachael-alexander.com

CHAPTER 1
STARTING COLLEGE OR UNIVERSITY

....

What would life be like if we had no courage to attempt anything?

Vincent Van Gogh

SCENARIO

....

Jack stalked out of the living room, slamming the door behind him.
Feeling angry but not really knowing why, he stormed into his
bedroom and stared with dismay at the multitude of boxes piled up
around him. Knowing the boxes' contents were furnishings for his room
at the university he was due to start, he felt the familiar sense of nausea
rising and the slow ache of stomach cramps starting.

It had all seemed such an exciting adventure when he had visited the
university campus back in April, but now the excitement had dissipated
and all he felt was a sense of dread and worry which seemed to have
been plaguing him for weeks. His state of mind was made worse by the
constant commentary by his well-meaning family, '*Ooh it won't be long
before you go now Jack*' and '*I bet you are really looking forward to
university Jack*'. He would plaster a smile on his face and nod his head
feigning enthusiasm, but underneath this mask, he was starting to panic
that going to university was the biggest mistake of his life. As freshers'
week drew nearer, he grew less and less enthusiastic about the whole
experience but couldn't tell anyone how he was truly feeling in case they
thought he was weak and stupid.

And now this morning he had struggled to catch his breath and the
gripping stomach pains had elevated to a new level. He really thought
there was something seriously wrong with him and had even started
to imagine terrible things would happen to his family when he left
for university. He would busy himself to distract himself from these
thoughts, but they plagued him incessantly, especially in the evenings.

He didn't want to worry his mum by telling her he was having second thoughts as he could see she had her own worries caused by a particularly stressful time at work. Also, he had seen how much money she had spent on bedding, lamps and kitchen equipment for his new life and didn't want this to be wasted. Feeling exhausted, Jack put his headphones in, pulled his hood up and distracted himself with social media: he had learned long ago that avoidance was the best way of blocking out intrusive thoughts and feelings.

Remember ... you've got this

It is understandable Jack is having these thoughts and feelings. You see, as humans, we prefer the familiar; we like routines, habits and structure in our lives and Jack is operating in his comfort zone in his current life. The thought of leaving the familiar and going to university can be scary as it is the unknown. His current life makes Jack feel emotionally *safe* as he knows he is not at risk of being hurt physically, emotionally or mentally. This is why many people do not like change – because change brings uncertainty which is scary. Yet, think about how this scenario might play out. By moving out of his comfort zone through facing his fears and starting university Jack can learn that new beginnings can feel scary, and it is perfectly normal to have doubts and even anxiety.

When your future appears uncertain, your internal hardwiring triggers a protective alarm response called fear, and hormones such as adrenaline and cortisol are released into your bloodstream. These hormones can make you feel a certain way and for good reason – to make you stop and reflect on whether the experience you are considering is safe and how likely you are to survive it. This is how the human race has survived for so many years.

However, because this biological chemical response can make you feel nauseous and short of breath and give you an impending sense of doom, you may retreat into what you perceive as safety and don't embrace the new experience. You stay stuck in your comfort zone. Sadly, life can then feel meaningless, and you may start to display behavioural symptoms called depression where you question the meaning of your life and not achieving your soul potential.

As Jack has never left home and moved to university before, he has no actual evidence of whether he will feel safe and be able to handle university meaning he is unable to feel calm at this moment in time. His worry is triggering his fear response, meaning adrenaline and cortisol are consistently being released into his bloodstream, causing biological symptoms of nausea and stomach cramps to continue. This in turn increases the amount of worry he experiences which in turn triggers more hormones to be released and the cycle continues. The medical model calls this anxiety, yet, in reality, it is simply a biological fear response out of control which Jack has never been taught how to control. Social media scrolling is simply a distraction technique, trying to block out his fearful thoughts. The best action for Jack to take is to use his courage to power through his fears by talking to someone about how he feels and he will realise how he feels is an expected response when dealing with change.

Understandably, there may be times when you feel so emotionally overwhelmed that you choose, or are advised to take, psychiatric medication to help you cope and this may be the right thing to do. While it takes great courage to admit you are struggling with uncomfortable physiological symptoms such as low mood, medication does not always help you face the core fears and limiting beliefs which are causing you to feel overwhelmed. All your emotions, both the positive and not so positive, are valuable signposts to guide you through your life. The more you realise you can handle anything which comes your way, including your emotions, the more you can live a happy and successful life. The strategies in this book will help you learn how to do this.

TOPIC 1.1 I HAVE CHANGED MY MIND AND I DON'T WANT TO GO TO UNIVERSITY

Well done, it takes great courage to change your mind and you should be very proud of yourself! Since making the decision to attend university, you may have realised something about yourself or your life which means you want to choose a different option, and this is okay. Maybe you felt pressurised to go but have now realised university is not your preferred option. Awesome!

However, sometimes you may want to change your mind, but in reality, it is fear making you doubt your original choice. A new experience, one you haven't conquered before, can appear scary, meaning you try to avoid it as you think you may fail or are unable to handle it in some way. It is understandable you may have doubts right now about leaving home and going to university as it is a huge step into the unknown. However, it is well known that if students stick at university for the first six weeks, they'll normally see their course through to the end as it can take those six weeks for you to adjust to the new environment.

You may currently be feeling out of control as you are not sure what is going to happen at university. You may think you will struggle with the workload, fail to make new friends, miss home or even that you will be miserable for the next three years. While these worries are natural, in reality, these events are unlikely to happen, and you don't want your fear to stop you from embarking on a potentially life-changing experience.

The interesting component about fear is once you have faced your fear, your worries disappear. So perhaps you would rather look back in six months and be able to say, '*I had my doubts about going to university, but I felt the fear and did it anyway and it is an amazing experience*'. Equally, you may say '*I am so proud of myself because I tried university and I found out it wasn't for me*'.

Either way, you win as you have shown yourself how brave you really were by facing your fears. And if you really have changed your mind, then yes, some people around you will probably freak out for a few days, but they will get over it once they realise you have a right to make a different decision to what they want or what you once wanted, which is all part of maturing into an independent adult. Well done.

SELF-ENQUIRY REFLECTION 1.1

So, let's recap. Yes, you can change your mind (even if others will freak out) but make sure it isn't your fear which is tricking you into thinking you don't want to go to university. Remember, you have a right to admit you are scared – being scared is part of being human.

I have the courage to admit I feel scared.

1. On a scale of 0–10 (10 being *you've got this*) how do I feel about going to university?

2. What specific doubts and worries do I have about going to university?

Remember, it is completely understandable and acceptable to have these doubts because university is a new experience.

3. What would I say to a friend who was having these doubts and worries?

4. What am I looking forward to regarding the university experience?

5. If I acted with courage, what would my choice be?

LIFE LESSON

It is perfectly acceptable to change your mind in life; however, you must ensure fear is not trying to change your mind for you. The more you face your fears and embrace new opportunities in your life, the more confident you will feel and the less anxiety you will experience. Avoidance of exciting new experiences and opportunities can make life very dull indeed.

TOPIC 1.2 I WANT TO QUIT AND GO HOME

For every student who loves the university experience, there is one who doesn't and of course, you have the right to leave university at any time. However, it is worth remembering that it can take time to adjust and adapt to any new life experience as you are transitioning through a time of change which can make you feel emotionally unsettled. Leaving adolescence can be hard and you are probably missing the old life you had; your friends, family, bedroom and maybe your family pet, so be kind to yourself.

In addition, university life can be extremely challenging at times, especially at the beginning. You may feel exhausted by the newness of it all and feel like you want to give up and go home. But remember how brave you have been to get this far – leaving the safety of your own home and learning to stand on your own two feet; what an achievement.

Of course, you may have valid reasons for wanting to go home. You may think you don't understand your subject, or feel like you don't know what you are doing and everybody else on your course seems to get it but of course they don't.

Perhaps you have realised you are fed up with studying and want to work instead. Something may have happened at home and you want to return to support others. It may even be as simple as realising that university life is not what you thought, and this is okay too.

There could be all sorts of reasons you want to quit and have the courage to own these reasons. This means taking responsibility and admitting why you want to go home; but make sure your reasons are valid.

- Is it because you are struggling to get good grades because you are having too much fun (understandable) or because of your other commitments and responsibilities?
- Is it because you have struggled to make new friends because you have been missing friends from home and been online with them every night?
- Is it because you have no money, perhaps because you are struggling to manage your own finances for the first time?

Have the courage to take a step back and reflect on how you can improve your situation as this is an empowering act and a sign of maturity, intelligence and wisdom.

SELF-ENQUIRY REFLECTION 1.2

....

Do you really want to go home or are you simply feeling overwhelmed with how different university is from school and college? Remember, you are going through change, and it can take time to adjust to Higher Education. Your answers to these questions will help you explore your thoughts and help empower yourself to make the right decision.

I have the courage to end something I am not enjoying.

1. On a scale of 0–10 (10 being the maximum) how much do I want to go home right now?

2. What are my reasons and how valid are these reasons to me?

Remember to reach out to people who can provide insight to help you make your decision (personal tutor, lecturer, friend, parent, relative, counsellor, internet). If you want to leave, then this is okay but leave for the right reasons.

3. If I decide to stay, how can I commit 100 per cent to my university experience; what action can I take to improve it?

4. Who else can support me in improving my experience while I am here? (*personal tutor, lecturer, friend, parent, relative, counsellor, internet*)

5. If I acted with courage, what choice would I make?

LIFE LESSON

....

It is perfectly acceptable to end something, but, first, ensure you are not self-sabotaging a potentially successful outcome. By committing your time, focus and energy 100 per cent you may be able to change your current experience. If you commit to making your experience as good as it can be, the more empowered you will feel.

TOPIC 1.3 I THINK I AM ON THE WRONG COURSE/AT THE WRONG UNIVERSITY

Students often want to change their course and/or university, so don't worry, you are not the first and won't be the last.

You may have made your course or university choice based on a limited amount of knowledge, for example after a short tour around the campus and a read of the course prospectus, but your real-life experience may be very different from your expectations.

In life, there are times when your expectations are not met, and this is okay. Experiencing disappointment is part of life and you should not berate yourself as wrong or stupid for making your original choice. You made it with the resources, feelings and knowledge you had available at the time so be kind to yourself. However, what's important is that you understand you can change your mind which means taking action to rectify the situation – which will not resolve itself.

Action you could take is to reach out for advice to help you make a more informed choice regarding the suitability of a different course and/or university. For example, it may be prudent to ask your current lecturer about future course content as it may just be the current content you are not enjoying. It also may be wise to have a chat with your personal tutor as he or she will have plenty of experience with this situation. If your current university facilities are not as you hoped, you could research another university to see if it suits your needs better. Once you have started to research your options, you will start to feel more empowered and back in control of the situation.

However, you do have to exercise caution as you may think another option will make you happier, yet it may not. It is common for people to have '*magical thinking*' which is believing another situation will make you happier based on no evidence whatsoever. However, you can increase the likelihood of an improved outcome if you fully research all your options.

There may be some people around you who do not believe it is the right thing for you to change your mind. However, this could be their fear as they may never have been encouraged to change their mind as a young person. Part of maturing is learning to trust your gut feelings or your heart, so believe you have a right to explore different options – after all this is your future, not theirs. You can always explore options which may help you realise you have made the right choice after all. At least you will feel more settled and able to commit to your current studies.

SELF-ENQUIRY REFLECTION 1.3

....

It takes courage to research alternative choices. This research will clarify the reasons you want to change your current situation and help you identify different options. It can be scary to change your mind after making a decision but the more you learn to do it, the easier it becomes.

I have the courage to research other options.

1. What are the reasons I want to change my course/university?

2. Looking at these reasons, how valid are they to *me*?
   (*Other people may have different views regarding the validity but please trust your own thoughts and feelings*)

3. What research can I undertake to explore my different options including who can I talk to who is *unbiased* to help me decide?
   (*Personal tutor, lecturer, friend, relative, internet, counsellor, parent*)

4. What benefits would changing my course/university give me?

5. What is the action I have to take to get the outcome I want?

LIFE LESSON

....

It is perfectly acceptable to explore different options in life, however, conducting as much research as possible will help you to make the most empowered decision. Remember to also learn to trust your gut feelings – your intuition. How you feel about something can often be more important than logical reasoning, but ensure fear is not making your choice for you.

TOPIC 1.4 I AM HOMESICK AND FEEL LONELY

The majority of new students would admit to feeling homesick at the start of their university experience. Feeling this way doesn't mean you are weak or acting like a child, it simply means you are experiencing the uncertainty and discomfort of transitioning from one part of your life to another. When you leave an environment, such as your home which feels familiar, and move somewhere new, it can feel scary because it is the unknown – you do not know what is going to happen and you can feel out of control. Therefore, you may crave the familiarity of the old environment. The most important thing is to not judge yourself negatively in any way but to tell yourself it is okay to feel exactly the way you do at this moment and that these feelings are likely to pass in time.

Often, you can feel homesick due to feeling lonely and it can take time to find a new friendship group when starting university. A good method of dealing with loneliness is to write down why you feel lonely and what you are specifically missing from your old life. This can help give you clarity as to why you are feeling homesick. From this, you may realise you are missing being part of a tribe, such as your old school/college friends or simply missing a particular family member.

However, it is important to believe, that in time you are likely to adjust and adapt to your new environment and routine, and your lonely feelings will dissipate. You will spend less time thinking about your old life as you become more fully engaged in your new life and learn to take responsibility in creating your new life.

You may be surrounded by people who are not missing home or who don't feel as lonely as you and this is perfectly acceptable and does not mean you are wrong in any way. It can simply mean you may have had a stronger support network at home who you are missing more or are taking slightly more time to adjust. There is no time limit on adapting to change, but if you feel the same way for a continued duration, it may be a good idea to have a chat with your tutor to see what additional support they can offer you.

If you are still feeling lonely or homesick after a longer duration, it may simply be that your new environment is not suiting you as an individual, and this is okay. Knowing when to let go of something is just as important as committing to something. It may be you would prefer to switch to the university in your home time yet live in halls of residency, for example, or even live back at home. We are all different and should not compare ourselves to others.

SELF-ENQUIRY REFLECTION I.4

....

Feeling homesick and lonely, even when surrounded by people, is an acceptable and understandable way to feel. These questions will help you reflect on what it is you are missing from your old life and how you can start to integrate more into your new life.

I have the courage to feel how I feel.

1. On a scale of 0–10, (10 being the maximum), how homesick do I feel right now?

2. On a scale of 1–10 (10 being the maximum), how lonely do I feel right now?

3. What activities help me feel less lonely?

4. Whose company do I enjoy which makes me feel less lonely?

5. Who can I reach out to help me feel better at this moment in time? (*Personal tutor, lecturer, friend, parent, relative, counsellor, internet*)

LIFE LESSON

....

As you transition through different chapters in your life, give yourself time to let go of the old chapter. Acknowledge that letting go is a time of loss and change and it is therefore important to simply sit with how you feel as grief can take time to process. By slowly letting go of the old, you can start to embrace the new.

TOPIC 1.5 I THINK I DON'T DESERVE MY UNIVERSITY PLACE

When you are feeling pressure to be someone or achieve something in your life, it is common to experience 'imposter syndrome'. This is when you psychologically feel like a phony, that you are going to be found out as a fraud and that you shouldn't be where you are – such as studying at university. You may feel undeserving of your university place, believing you achieved it through luck and not your hard work, ability and talent. This insecurity can lead to an extreme lack of confidence resulting in feelings of self-doubt and anxiety.

Many adults in the workplace also suffer with the imposter syndrome and it is therefore essential that you learn to overcome it now. Continued suffering means you can over-prepare, procrastinate and struggle to enjoy life due to a deep fear of failure. You can also feel unworthy of any success that you have worked hard to achieve. However, once you recognise, you have been hijacked by imposter syndrome at university, there is action you can take to feel better.

First, make a list of all the reasons you were awarded your place at university. Then imagine someone who loves you, such as a friend whose opinion you trust. What would he or she say to help you believe you have a right to your university place?

Second, be realistic about failure: everybody fails at something, and you are at university to learn and a substantial part of learning is failing. It is how you respond to failure that is important – learn from it as opposed to condemning yourself. Some say fail stands for first attempt in learning. You wouldn't shout at a small child for falling off their bike when they learn to ride, you would encourage them to keep practising and the same is applicable for you.

Seek expertise if your self-doubt (the cause of imposter syndrome) is overwhelming you – speak to your lecturer or personal tutor to hear positive validation regarding your skills. If you are procrastinating on a piece of work, due to believing you can't do it, then break it down into small manageable goals. Commit to 15 minutes only and after 15 minutes give yourself permission to stop if you want. This reduces procrastination which is rooted in fear.

You are not alone in having self-doubt and many students struggle with imposter syndrome. However, the more you learn to believe and trust in your abilities, the quicker it will disappear, and you will enjoy your university experience much more and obtain the results you want and deserve.

SELF-ENQUIRY REFLECTION 1.5

. . . .

Imposter syndrome can be rooted in self-doubt and a lack of faith in your ability. These questions will help you self-validate, enabling you to be confident in your abilities.

I have the courage to own my magnificence.

1. On a scale of 0–10 (10 being the maximum) how much do I suffer with imposter syndrome?

2. Why do I think you struggle with imposter syndrome?
   (*Reflect on if you have always struggled with it in your life. Have you ever been given positive validation throughout your life?*)

3. List at least three reasons why I am deserving of my current success.

4. How will I stop the imposter syndrome from negatively affecting my university experience?

5. What action can I take to get over my fear of failure and procrastination?

LIFE LESSON

. . . .

Many people struggle with a fear of failure, meaning they may not start anything new in their life. However, if you believe there is no such thing as failure, only an opportunity to learn something, then your fear of failure will disappear. You are good enough, so believe in your abilities, and enjoy the success you deserve.

TOPIC 1.6 I AM MISSING MY FAMILY/PETS/FRIENDS/PLACES

....

When you live somewhere which feels familiar, you can feel part of a tribe which gives you a sense of belonging. However, when you leave familiar people and places, you can feel sad, lonely, at risk and therefore vulnerable. These feelings can make you feel overwhelmed which can make you want to cry. Although being upset may appear to add to your negative state of mind, is it essential as it simply means you are acknowledging a loss of something.

You may have cravings to go back home to familiar routines and people that you know. You may even be questioning if you have made the right decision attending university or starting to worry you have made the wrong course choice. This doubt can come from craving the familiar and as your university experience is new, you are still in the unfamiliar which is causing worry. But remember as the new becomes more familiar, uncertainty will pass, you will start to feel more confident and miss home less and less.

Have compassion for yourself as you journey through this major life change and buy some tissues to have a good cry-athon. Once you feel a little better, reflect on how you can fully commit to this new chapter in your life. Perhaps you can ask a friend if they want to go for a walk or you can go to the library to find a positive self-help book. Always focus on the future, not the past and remind yourself why you came to university. By setting small goals to embrace the present moment, you are making your university experience the best it can be. Sitting in your room, face timing your pet spaniel every evening is not going to help you enjoy your university experience or get the grade that you deserve.

If after a few weeks, you feel no better, reach out to a professional such as your tutor. Remember you will not be the first student to miss home and simply expressing how you feel is beneficial for your mental health. Also hearing from your tutor that how you feel is a normal reaction to first-year student life will also help you feel better. It is normal to feel sad and cry when you leave things that you love behind, yet committing to your new life shows courage and maturity.

SELF-ENQUIRY REFLECTION I.6

. . . .

These questions will help you analyse what you are missing from your old life, giving you an increased awareness of why you feel the way you do. Letting go of your old life and moving on is a great way to experience new opportunities and live life to the full.

I have the courage to let go of the old and embrace my new life.

1. On a scale of 0–10 (10 being the maximum) how much am I missing home?

2. What specifically am I missing from my previous life at home? (*ie, company, familiar faces, pet, love, encouragement, fun*)

3. How can I bring the elements I am missing from home into my new life here?

4. How am I spending more time focused on the past than planning my amazing future?

5. How can I commit to ensuring my university experience is as awesome as I deserve it to be? (*Think about who you can speak to who may be able to help you*)

LIFE LESSON

. . . .

Being human means, you experience loss and miss things that you love which makes you cry. This is called grief. Remember, it takes courage to have new experiences, meet new people and enjoy new places but when you do this, you reap the rewards as you become more confident and secure in your ability to handle loss and change throughout your life.

TOPIC 1.7 I FEEL LIKE I DON'T FIT IN

....

It can be upsetting when you leave old friendship groups as you may struggle to immediately fit into a new one. Not fitting in can make you feel isolated, lonely and different from the majority in some way, leading to feelings of being the 'odd one out'. A natural response when you don't fit in is to think, 'there must be something wrong with me', especially when it seems others fit in so effortlessly. Thinking this can make you doubt yourself, as though you are inadequate or flawed in some way.

Yet there is nothing inadequate about you, as you are unique which is a beautiful thing indeed. It is understandable you want to fit in but before you try too hard to fit in, ask yourself, 'What group am I trying to fit in with and are they like me in any way at all'? This means asking yourself if they think, feel and behave in similar ways to you.

It is understandable that you want to be part of a bigger group simply to feel accepted and that you belong somewhere. However, there is nothing lonelier than being part of a group where you have nothing in common or you have to change yourself to be more like the majority. Instead of asking yourself do they like me, try asking yourself, do I like them?

It takes confidence and courage to be yourself and accept the way you think and feel, even if it is different from the majority. You may have been raised differently from others and because of this, you may have a different mindset and way of seeing the world. This can make you feel like you don't fit in, but this certainly doesn't mean you are flawed in any way, simply that you have been raised to view life differently. Alternatively, you may be shy, quite sensitive and quite rightly, it takes time for you to trust people, meaning it takes longer for you to find the right friendship group. Meanwhile, it is important you celebrate your uniqueness and know that you are good enough exactly as you are.

Your journey through life is one of finding people who have a similar vibe to you, those whose company you enjoy. This is known as '*finding your tribe*' and sometimes it takes time. However, in the meantime being able to enjoy your own company is a sign of courage. Of course, it is great to have friends and companionship, but only if these people add joy, inspiration, happiness and fun into your life. The more you are your authentic self, the more you will attract similar people to you – have patience; it will happen.

SELF-ENQUIRY REFLECTION 1.7

....

These questions will help you identify why you feel like you don't fit in, but more importantly what group of people you would like to fit in with. The important part of fitting in is realising being your real authentic self is more important than trying to fit in with people who are unlike you.

I have the courage to be myself.

1. On a scale of 0–10 of fitting in (10 being the maximum), how much do I feel like I fit in?

2. Why do I feel like I don't fit in?

3. If I did fit in, what would be different in my life?

4. How will I know when I have found my tribe – what will we have in common?

5. What action can I take to find this person or group of people?

LIFE LESSON

....

Your tribe should be one that helps you become a better person – helping you evolve psychologically, emotionally and spiritually. You deserve to be surrounded by people who have your best interests at heart. When you are not afraid of your own company you can be more selective about who you want to spend your time with meaning you create very special relationships.

TOPIC 1.8 I AM STRUGGLING TO MAKE FRIENDS

As you grow older, you can become increasingly self-conscious, and it can become harder to make new friends. As you neurologically develop, you can start to fear being rejected, disapproved of and even not being liked. Your self-doubt can make you wonder if others will like you and want to spend time with you. Because of this fear of rejection, you can self-sabotage when it comes to making new friends, thinking you are better off alone and you may withdraw into yourself. Life can then feel really lonely.

However, one thing many students have in common is being new to the university environment and have left friends from school or college behind. Therefore, most students are looking to make friends to help make the university experience more fun and meaningful! Of course, it is easy to stay in touch with old friends virtually through using social media, however, making new friends is great too. The hardest part of making new friends is reaching out to others because you are risking rejection which can feel scary and painful. However, what is more scary and painful is being alone without like-minded friends to share this new experience. So, face your fears, draw on your courage and reach out to others.

Of course, there may be a little voice in your head saying, 'What if they don't want to be friends with me?' Ask yourself, why wouldn't they want to be friends with me? You are interesting and interested, articulate, thoughtful, kind and sincere, meaning you are great company to be with. You have been a good friend to others in the past and you can do it again. It is time to realise the gift you are to others and how you make a positive difference to their lives.

Your energy system (how you feel) attracts people to you who have a similar energy, so become aware of those whom you feel comfortable with. Next, reach out to them by simply making conversation about anything at all. Remember they are probably feeling as scared as you are so will be grateful you had the courage to initiate the conversation. It takes time to build a friendship, but you can do this – just one small step out of your comfort zone.

The key to great friendships is quality not quantity. Having one friend who you trust and you can be yourself with is more beneficial than having a large group of friends who you fear are talking negatively about you. Friendship is caring about each other, knowing you would have each other's back when life gets tough sometimes. It is okay if it takes you time to meet the right friend – the universe will guide you in this of course.

SELF-ENQUIRY REFLECTION 1.8

....

It can be a challenge to make new friends and these questions will help you understand the type of friend you want, meaning you will have a better chance of being part of a solid, empowering friendship group.

I have the courage to make new friends.

1. On a scale of 0–10 (10 being the maximum), how much do I think I am struggling to make new friends?

2. As a friend, what do I offer to another?

3. What are the qualities I would like in a friend?

4. If I were feeling brave, what action could I take to reach out to others?

5. If a friend from my past or anyone who knows me gave me a testimonial about me as a friend – what do I think they would say?

Some people think that having lots of friends is a sign of how popular they are, yet often just having one or two close friends can be so much more satisfying. Quality over quantity.

LIFE LESSON

....

As you transition through life, the ability to make new friends is important, as friends can make a challenging day better. When you truly believe you are a good friend, you can pick and choose who you want to be friends with as you know you have a lot to offer another. It is important to know what a good friendship looks like in order that you are truly supported.

TOPIC 1.9 I DON'T KNOW WHETHER TO FIND A PART-TIME JOB OR VOLUNTEER MY TIME

Part of the university experience is learning to to make decisions. One of the decisions you may have to make is whether to find work and/or volunteer. Of course, adjusting to the university experience may take time initially so you may decide not to do this immediately or circumstances may mean you have to find work quickly to help finance your way. Whatever your circumstances, there are many benefits to working part time whether it be paid work or volunteering.

Like a lot of university experiences, finding work may be out of your comfort zone and this means it can feel scary. When you feel overwhelmed, it is easy to put your head in the sand and not take action, simply because you don't know where to start. However, if finding work is a necessity or volunteering will help your job prospects, then finding ways to get over these feelings is important.

Finding work can build your confidence. Confidence is when you face your fears and therefore take action to go after what you want in life. Working is valuable as it helps you become more confident as you learn you can handle new experiences. Of course, the other benefit is having financial independence and the freedom to spend and save money.

The first step in finding work is taking time to consider where you would like to work and how many hours you would like to work. Then identify if these places are recruiting. A quick search online or contacting the venue will give you the answer. Each vacancy may have a different recruitment procedure so research what the organisation wants – is it a curriculum vitae (CV) or online application procedure? Your tutor may also be able to help you find opportunities due to their local connections or even give you help in writing your CV.

The one thing which could be stopping you from finding work is you; thinking that you are not qualified or suitable in any way. This is your self-doubt and, like discussed above, the only way to disprove this incorrect thinking is to apply. Of course, you may not get the first job or placement you go after, but don't let this stop you. You will be the right fit for the right place – trust in the universe to deliver.

SELF-ENQUIRY REFLECTION 1.9

....

Deciding whether to work or volunteer is a choice you may have to make at university. These questions will help you understand if fear is stopping you from making the right decision regarding finding work and/ or volunteering. Remember both activities are a great way to build your social confidence.

I have the courage to explore work or volunteering opportunities.

1. What would be the benefits of working or volunteering?

2. What would be the benefits of *not* working or volunteering?

3. What may be stopping me from finding work or a volunteering placement?

4. Identify if these are excuses or fear. (*ie, you may say you haven't got time, but is this really a fear of rejection if you don't get the job?*)

5. What action can I take to find work or a volunteering placement?

LIFE LESSON

....

The more confident you can become in applying for and starting new jobs, the more opportunities you will have as you progress through life. As people get older, many tend to stay in unfulfilling jobs even though they are unhappy as they are afraid of leaving what is familiar. However, by getting over your fears of this now, you will be a gift to any employer and will always do work you love as you journey through life.

CHAPTER 2
UNDERSTANDING AND MANAGING RELATIONSHIPS

··

The most exciting, challenging, and significant relationship of all is the one you have with yourself. And, if you find someone to love the you that you love, well, that's just fabulous

Carrie Bradshaw SITC TV show

SCENARIO

················

Ronan groaned as he realised he still hadn't let his mum know the date he would be arriving home for the Christmas holiday. The thought of having to spend three weeks at home playing *happy families* was making him feel anxious. He didn't dislike his parents, in fact, he loved hanging out with them individually, but the constant arguments they had with each other created an unbearably tense atmosphere at home. Even from a young age, he had been confused about why they had stayed together and had even been secretly jealous of his friend Tom who seemed a lot happier when his parents divorced.

From being seven years old Ronan had witnessed arguments and silent feuds between his parents. He and his older sister Adele had constantly felt stuck in the middle, having to take sides to defend either one of them or trying to get them to be nice to each other.

Ronan had experienced years of hurt and felt deep pain when either one of his parents would shout they were leaving the other and he would cry himself to sleep, fearing being left alone as the front door slammed shut as one parent stormed out. Yet a few days later, mum or dad would return like nothing had happened and a sense of calmness would remain for a few weeks. Each time Ronan would think everything was going to be okay, then the arguments and abusive cycle would start all over again.

Because of his past, Ronan couldn't understand why anyone would ever get married as it seemed one long argument or resentment-filled feud. Ronan perceived marriage as a trap and had made a silent vow to never be put in that position, especially after Adele had just announced she was divorcing for the second time.

Ronan had experienced a few relationships since he was 15 but always ended it when he felt the girl wanted more from him. He liked to be in control of the pace of the relationship and would refer to his partners as simply *friends who are girls* as giving them the title of *girlfriend* felt too serious. This made him feel safe as he didn't want to get too close, potentially putting himself at risk of feeling the same pain he experienced as a child. Most of the girls seemed to be ok with this and if they weren't, they were cut loose.

Ronan thought about the girl he was seeing now, Sofia. Even though he was being a bit distant, there was something different about her which intrigued him. She didn't seem as needy as girls from his past and had her own interests and friendship group. She never seemed to put pressure on him and if he couldn't see her, she didn't seem to nag or moan at him like the other girls used to. She never harassed him about the status of their relationship, such as asking if they were *exclusive* and seemed to just enjoy his company. She also talked about her future and her ambitions which he found attractive.

Ronan sighed, knowing he really needed to confirm his plans to his mum. He looked online and checked the university timetable again to confirm the date the semester ended. He briefly wondered about inviting Sofia to his parents for Christmas, but then not wanting her to witness the bad atmosphere, he quickly decided against it.

....

Remember ... you've got this

The relationships you witnessed in your childhood can affect how harmonious your adult relationships are. For example, you may have witnessed a non-loving marriage between your parents or those who cared for you, such as your grandparents. You may have been raised by someone who was suffering from an addiction which meant they showed a lack of love to you. You may have even been raised in the care system which means although you may have felt loved, you may have felt rejected as a child.

Sadly, some of these experiences may have resulted in you not recognising healthy loving behaviour being demonstrated to you. In addition, if you feel unworthy of being shown love in anyway because you were not made to feel loved in your childhood, this then affects the type of relationships you attract and accept. You may also struggle to show yourself love and respect.

Once you become more aware of how relationships modelled to you as a child can affect your behaviour, the more you can start to make more powerful, conscious decisions. For example, Ronan is scared that committing to a relationship may cause him pain in the same way he saw his parents suffer. However, behaving in this way is potentially stopping him from experiencing a great connection with someone. Once he becomes aware that his past negative experience and current fear is controlling his choices, he can become more conscious and change his behaviour.

If you can learn to discern how loving or unloving people really are, you will experience positive relationships, whether this is a friendship or an intimate relationship. This is important because you may meet people who sadly do not realise, they are behaving in an unloving way, meaning your relationship will struggle, often mirroring what you experienced as a child.

You may have been raised to value physical attractiveness or how ambitious or how financially viable someone is, for example, rather than appreciating their inner values of kindness, empathy, resilience and humour. This can then mean that when challenging times occur, there is a lack of support due to your partner not knowing how to protect, nurture and love you. Alternatively, you may have been raised to be a people pleaser and rescuer, meaning you want to fix, rescue or heal another which means you can quickly become drained of energy due to over-supporting another and therefore your well-being becomes affected.

Sometimes, you may feel pressure to find that one special relationship which will make you feel loved, yet you need to feel good enough and love yourself first. While it can be fulfilling to meet that special someone you want to spend your life with, experiencing different intimate relationships at different times in your life can help you understand the type of person you want to be and the type of person you want to be with.

UNDERSTANDING AND MANAGING RELATIONSHIPS

Ultimately, the spiritual aim of any relationship is to help you love and respect yourself unconditionally. This may be through someone treating you in a disrespectful way, where you end the connection because you realise you are worthy of being treated better. Or preferably you find someone who can demonstrate love and respect to you as they appreciate how lucky they are to have you in their life.

Always ask yourself how a connection is helping you be a better person and have the courage to consider leaving any relationship which is not enabling you to achieve this.

TOPIC 2.1 I AM WORRIED MY RELATIONSHIP WILL END WHEN I LEAVE FOR UNIVERSITY

You may be concerned that your current relationship will end when you leave for university and the thought of this may be filling you with dread. However, it is important to believe your relationship can survive while you are at university, as plenty do. It is also important you do not let this fear stop you from enjoying your university experience. Relationships can often become stronger through a period of absence, especially if they have strong foundations, and modern technology will help you keep in touch with your loved one while you are away.

To ensure you give your relationship the best chance of survival consider the following tips.

- Always aim for open and honest communication with your partner, no matter how scared these conversations may make you feel.
- Be aware online messaging can be ambiguous and unclear so opt for having face-to-face conversations as much as you can.
- If you see yourself exhibiting controlling or needy behaviour, perhaps out of fear, reflect on why you are behaving this way and be open with your partner about how you feel. If your partner behaves in this way, reflect back to him or her what you are experiencing and how it makes you feel.
- Be clear on your boundaries – for example, how often will you see each other or speak to each other in order for your relationship to flourish. However, recognise these boundaries may change as you both adapt to the new circumstances.
- Try to avoid drunk texting or talking as this can often end badly.
- If you get fearful that your relationship will end, trust that the right outcome will occur. Some relationships are destined to be life-partner relationships from a young age and yours could well be one of these.

Use your university experience to help define the type of relationship you want to be in and if your relationship shifts from one of joy, contentment and happiness to one of pain, arguments and unhappiness then it is a sure sign to let it go and move on.

SELF-ENQUIRY REFLECTION 2.1

....

Life can be about experiencing love with many different people in your life and not everyone settles at a young age. However, these questions will help you ensure your current relationship flourishes rather than falters.

I have the courage to trust in my relationship.

1. What are my top three concerns about being in a long-distance relationship?

2. What evidence do I have the concerns listed above will actually happen?

3. What challenges could arise in our relationship while I am away at university?

4. How can we both prevent these from happening?

5. What action do we both need to take to ensure our relationship has the best chance of flourishing?

LIFE LESSON

....

When you are in a relationship, if both parties set the intention of growing to be more self-aware, spiritually evolved and happier then this ensures the relationship will be a healthy one. Some relationships do have an expiry date and having the courage to let go means you can find solace alone or in a happier relationship.

TOPIC 2.2 I AM STRUGGLING TO FIND A NEW RELATIONSHIP

It is natural to want to share your life experience with someone; however, it is important that your relationship adds joy and happiness to your life rather than anxiety and worry. Some people settle and accept an unloving, even toxic, relationship as they have sub-conscious fears about being alone or feeling unlovable. Yet it takes courage and strength to find a relationship which develops you both as individuals.

While you are single, use the time to think about the type of person you want to be with and the type of relationship you want to be in. Great relationships connect on multiple levels.

- Physically – you find each other attractive, wanting to be intimate with each other and there is strong chemistry between you both.
- Mentally – you stimulate, challenge and engage each another to think in an empowering way, helping each other to become more aware of yourself and life.
- Emotionally – you can show your true emotions and be vulnerable in sharing your thoughts of how you really feel.
- Spiritually – you encourage each other to be a more loving person through self-awareness, honesty, trust and compassion, helping each other find purpose, passion and meaning in life.

Being in a new relationship can be exciting; however, you may feel pressurised to find 'the one' – the person you want to stay with for the rest of your life. However, this can be an idea from fairy tales you may have been read as a child and may not be right for you. Different people are brought into your life to teach you awareness about yourself and life and these are not always long term. You may have a relationship which lasts three months which brings you more awareness of how lovable you are and the type of person you want to be than someone with whom you have a 25-year marriage.

When you are dating ask yourself these questions.

- Is this person interesting – do they keep me stimulated, mentally and emotionally?
- Is this person interested in me – do they ask me questions about me and my life and are they genuinely interested in the answers?
- Do they have a positive outlook on life, or are they negative in any way?
- How is their relationship with their parents – are they hurt, bitter or resentful in any way of their childhood?
- Do they encourage, inspire and listen to the goals you have set yourself?

- If you are having a bad day, do they listen and support you and vice versa?
- What chemical stimulants do they use to cope with life?

While these questions may seem obscure, the answers will help you discern if you have met a person who is able to look after your heart and not mess with your head. There is no such thing as perfection and relationships are about compromise, yet meeting someone who is kind, supportive and empathetic means they will support you and not sabotage you in life. You may be helping each other to heal which is a true spiritual connection.

SELF-ENQUIRY REFLECTION 2.2

....

You may not have been raised to think about the inner qualities someone has. For example, it is more common to value someone's physical attributes than how kind they are. These questions will help you become clear about the type of person you want to be in a relationship with.

I have the courage to know what I want in a relationship.

1. On a scale of 0–10 (10 being the maximum), how important is it for me to connect with someone physically, mentally, emotionally and spiritually?

2. What are the inner qualities I would like someone to possess?
   (*eg, honesty, kindness, empathy, intelligence, emotional resilience*)

3. What are the inner qualities I currently possess?

4. What qualities and behaviours will I not tolerate from a partner?

5. What other research can I conduct to help ensure I am in a relationship which empowers me?
   (*eg, self-help books, social media, online courses, counsellor, coach, parent, friend*)

LIFE LESSON

....

There can be a great deal of pressure to find a life partner and settle down, but life can be about having many beautiful relationship experiences with different people. Take the pressure off yourself to find *the one* and allow the divine consciousness to link you with the right person at the right time.

TOPIC 2.3 HOW DO I KNOW IF MY RELATIONSHIP IS TOXIC, EVEN ABUSIVE?

....

Realising your relationship is toxic can be a harsh reality to face but it is better to be aware so you can make the choice to leave, rather than the relationship negatively affecting your mental health. The difficulty with recognising a toxic relationship is that the other person does not behave in an abusive way all the time and they have moments of treating you nicely. This can then make you feel on confused and on edge as you never know if the *nice* or *not so nice* partner is present.

Both men and women can be drawn in by a toxic partner but if a person truly loves you, they will not want to cause you physical, emotional or mental pain. However, some people, due to a neglectful childhood, are only able to prioritise their own needs which means your needs will always come second. This can mean your relationship will be one of conflict, tension and hostility a lot of the time.

There are many great resources on the internet to help you recognise toxic behaviour in others. If you think your relationship is one of control, demands, pressure, arguments and conflict then you may find these helpful. You may also like to explore the concept of trauma bonding.

If your partner behaves in any of the following ways, then you are in a toxic relationship.

- Expects you to give in to their demands constantly and will nag until you do.
- Is unable to compromise and will manipulate you until you give in.
- Will criticise, belittle and put you down, making you feel unworthy and like you constantly have to defend yourself.
- You walk on eggshells around them, so they don't erupt or sulk.
- You give in for a *quiet life*, to avoid sulking, tension and arguments.
- If you challenge their criticism of you, they will say you are '*being too sensitive*' or '*I'm only joking*' making you feel like the bad person.
- They will deny, sulk, ghost or block you if you try to call them out on their behaviour.
- They rarely take an interest in your day, unless it is from a position of wanting to know where you have been and who you have been with (control).
- They are grumpy, negative and complain about most things in life, nothing is ever good enough for them, including you.
- They rarely talk about the inner qualities they love in you and are more interested in how you benefit them and their lifestyle.
- They say they will change their behaviour, but the changed behaviour is never consistent, meaning you have the same arguments repeatedly.

You have a right to be happy and live free from this and deserve to be with someone who knows how to treat a person they love and respect.

SELF-ENQUIRY REFLECTION 2.3

....

I have the courage to be free from a toxic relationship.

1. On a scale of 0–10 (10 being the maximum), how much do I think I am in a toxic relationship?

2. How does this awareness make me feel?

If you feel any overwhelming emotion as you are answering these, please let it be released. Keep repeating 'I am safe' in your mind repeatedly. There are lots of people who can help you leave this relationship when you feel ready.

3. How does the thought of leaving the relationship make me feel?

Many people are scared to leave a toxic relationship as their self-worth has been diminished so it is important you show yourself lots of self-compassion at this time.

4. What other red flags have I experienced in my relationship which upsets me?

5. Who can I reach out to for support to help me deal with this realisation? (*parent, friend, tutor, external agency, internet resources, police*)

LIFE LESSON

....

Toxic relationships can be with a range of people – partners, colleagues, bosses, friends and even family. It is important to recognise toxic behaviour in order that you stay away from these people. When you have high levels of self-worth, you only spend time with people who care about you and not those who harm you.

TOPIC 2.4 I HAVE STARTED A RELATIONSHIP, BUT I FEEL ANXIOUS IT WILL END

....

While the start of a relationship can be exciting and exhilarating, it can also be a time of worry and apprehension, wondering how the other person really feels about you, and if the relationship has a future. If your partner occasionally seems distant, you may start to feel anxious as you do not want to lose the loving feelings you have been experiencing and may even think there is something unlovable or wrong with you. Checking your phone constantly to see if they have messages is a sign of being worried.

However, the person you are in a relationship with has a past which determines how they behave towards you in relationships. Researchers such as John Bowlby and Anna Freud have shown how your relationship with your primary caregiver as a child affects how you behave when you are in an adult relationship. *Attachment theory* helps you to understand not only your behaviour but that of the person you are in a relationship with, and you may like to explore this theory further.

An important element of any relationship is each of you wanting the other person to be happy. Sadly, some people only expect you to make their happiness a priority, but this is neither your job nor your responsibility. A new relationship is a fact-finding mission – witnessing how kindly the other person behaves towards you and if they have the emotional resilience to support themselves and be there for you. However, this applies to you too – are you able to support yourself emotionally and yet still able to support another?

Honest communication with each other is also key. Score yourself out of 10 (10 being the maximum) for the following statements.

1. I feel safe to share how I feel with my new partner.
2. I am supported emotionally by my partner.
3. I support my partner emotionally.
4. I can talk openly and honestly with my partner about how I feel.
5. My partner can talk honestly and openly with me about how they feel.

Relationships are about helping each other develop as an individual. If you or your partner are unable to score well on these questions, then you may need to be brave and ask yourself if this is the right relationship for you both or how can you learn to communicate better. Also, be aware of red flags which are ways your partner may behave which do not seem very loving. It is easy to overlook this behaviour but it is important you have the courage to recognise it.

SELF-ENQUIRY REFLECTION 2.4

....

I have the courage to let my relationship unfold as it should.

1. On a scale of 0–10 (10 being the maximum), how happy am I in my new relationship?

2. What brings me joy in the relationship?

3. What causes me pain in the relationship?

4. Is it the person who is bringing joy/pain or is it the relationship itself?

Have the ability to discern the difference between the two – the person may bring you joy but the status of the relationship may bring you pain as it may not be playing out the way you want it to.

5. Who can you talk to who can offer you an unbiased opinion about your relationship? (*friend, counsellor, coach, parent, tutor, therapist, internet*)

LIFE LESSON

....

All relationships can teach you many things, especially how to unconditionally love and respect yourself. You may be in a relationship to numb feelings of loneliness or insecurity which can make you attract or even stay in an unsuitable relationship, but if your relationship is empowering you, then trust that it is the right thing for you at this time.

TOPIC 2.5 I WANT TO END MY RELATIONSHIP BUT DON'T WANT TO HURT THE OTHER PERSON

Ending a relationship takes courage as few people like to emotionally wound themselves and another. If the other person does not want the relationship to end, it may be especially hard for you to finish it as you do not want to cause the other person pain. This can be due to a behaviour pattern of prioritising another's happiness over your own. If you are particularly empathetic this may be a pattern in your life, but the more you understand you have a right to be happy, the better choices you will make regarding ending relationships.

There are different ways to end a relationship and of course, the preferred way for many is face to face. However, this may not be right for you, and that is okay – you have a right to choose the best method for you. You will also have your own reasons for ending the relationship and you don't even have to give a reason to the other person if you don't want to. Sometimes you may not logically know why you want to end the relationship but simply feel it is the right choice and that is okay too.

You may have outgrown your relationship – signs include no longer wanting to be around the person, choosing to avoid their calls, feeling irritated when you see them, or you may have started to argue more. It is important to remember you have a right to end the relationship, whether you have met someone else or simply do not want to be with that person.

The other person may beg you to continue the relationship; however, it is important to remember why you are ending the relationship and stay strong. Once the other person knows you are serious about ending the relationship, they may become abusive and not leave you alone, constantly ringing and harassing you. This is a time to reach out for support such as contacting the police to ensure this bullying stops. You do not deserve to be treated this way, simply for wanting to end a relationship. Sometimes the person you are ending the relationship with may be so distraught that their mental health may struggle and they may tell you they are going to end their life. Some people genuinely feel this way but others sadly use this as a form of control. When it is used as the latter, it is called emotional manipulation and may make you feel like a bad person, even believing you shouldn't end the relationship. However you have every right to end a relationship, regardless of how the other person acts. If you need support in dealing with this, please reach out to someone who can help you.

If your relationship has not been as loving as you expected, remember that there are some wonderful people in this world, and you will meet one who loves and respects you.

SELF-ENQUIRY REFLECTION 2.5

....

I have the courage and right to end my relationship.

1. On a scale of 0–10 (10 being the maximum) how much do I want to end the relationship?

2. What are my reasons for wanting to end the relationship?

3. On a scale of 0–10 (10 being the maximum) how much do I feel I have a right to end the relationship?

4. What are my fears about ending my relationship?

5. Who could I talk to if I need more support in ending the relationship? (*friend, counsellor, tutor, coach, parent, internet resources*)

LIFE LESSON

....

Being able to end a relationship with compassion and care for yourself is important. It is okay to end a relationship, no matter how long you have been in it. While it can feel scary and overwhelming, it can be the most empowering decision you can make for yourself and the other person.

TOPIC 2.6 I AM HEARTBROKEN AS MY RELATIONSHIP HAS ENDED

If your relationship has ended and it wasn't your choice (and even if it was), then you may experience a pain you have never experienced before. The feeling of grief which the loss can cause can feel like a physical pain which will never end.

It is understandable you may cry a lot and not want to see anyone or participate in any events. You may even become obsessed with your ex and want to find out as much as you can about his or her future. You may feel like you will never enjoy life again; however, your soul will heal in time, and there are some things you can do to help yourself.

- Spend time surrounded by those who do love and nurture you.
- Explain to people you may get upset and may cry sometimes and this is ok.
- Ignore those who say, 'get over it' as they cannot relate to the pain you feel.
- Reassure yourself that if the relationship is meant to be, then you will be together.
- Reflect on what you have learned about yourself and others by being in the relationship – how can you make your next relationship more harmonious?
- Try not to over-analyse what your ex is thinking as it is a waste of your valuable energy.
- Find activities which stimulate you and make your future better.
- Learn to show love and respect to yourself – explore what this means to you.
- If you want to heal by having duvet days and crying, then allow yourself.
- Consider seeing a counsellor or spiritual healer such as an astrologer or psychic to understand why the relationship ended.
- Keep your heart open and try not to become bitter or angry because of this experience.

In time your feelings will dissipate, and you will heal, although it may not feel like it now. You may look back and realise it was a love affair that helped you learn about love, yourself and relationships. The more love you felt, the more intense your heartbreak may feel. However, handling this depth of pain teaches you that you are stronger than you think, and this inner resilience means you will no longer fear opening your heart to another again as you know you can get over heartbreak. Remember, love doesn't hurt you, people demonstrating unloving behaviour do.

SELF-ENQUIRY REFLECTION 2.6

....

I have the courage to experience heartbreak.

1. On a scale of 0–10 (10 being the maximum) how much am I experiencing heartbreak right now?

The emotional pain of heartbreak can feel overwhelming at times, but crying will help you release your pain. However, if you feel suicidal, are self-harming, or using unhealthy coping mechanisms, please reach out to a professional for help.

2. What am I missing about my ex?

3. What am I missing about being in a relationship?

Is it your ex you are missing or the relationship or both? Sometimes you may think you are missing the person, but you are missing the connection rather than the qualities and traits of the person.

4. What have I learned about myself, love and relationships?

5. What different modalities of healing could I explore to help me heal? (*counselling, reiki healing, psychic readers, astrology readings, coach*)

LIFE LESSON

....

To experience love is to potentially experience heartbreak; however, this is no reason to not open your heart. Heartbreak is simply the soul grieving for a connection it once had and in time you may reconnect or love another. Knowing you can handle these deep feelings of pain means you have the inner-strength to handle anything which happens to you in your life.

TOPIC 2.7 I AM SINGLE, AND ALL MY FRIENDS ARE IN RELATIONSHIPS

....

Single life can be perceived as painful as you may feel lonely or be judging yourself negatively, believing there is something wrong with you because you don't have a partner. You may even stay in a relationship to avoid being alone or because you think you won't ever meet anyone else; however, this can mean you are settling for less than you deserve. In reality, being single can be an act of empowerment and bravery as you realise you are strong enough to handle life alone, learning to independently meet your needs while you wait for someone who truly adds love, joy and happiness into your life.

The attitude of others may also make you feel like you are failing in some way, being asked questions such as, don't you have a partner? or are you still single? This line of questioning can make you feel as though there is something wrong with you, yet it is an act of autonomy to stand alone, knowing you do not need anyone else to make you happy.

There are many benefits to being single such as:

- you become more confident as you learn to meet your own physical, emotional, mental and spiritual needs;
- you realise you are independent not having to rely on anyone else;
- you can choose to do what you want to do when you want to do it;
- you can socialise with whomever you want, whenever you want;
- you have freedom and flexibility to be spontaneous each day;
- you do not have to compromise with another in any way;
- you can plan your future the way you want it;
- you can accept invitations without having to check with someone else;
- you can spend time focusing on your personal and spiritual development;
- you can go on dates, learning what you want in a future partner;
- you avoid arguments or tensions which arise in any relationship;
- you do not have another's emotions or problems affecting your life.

Of course, you will have moments of feeling alone or lonely; however, these times do pass, and you can reach out to other people in your life for nurture, love and social contact. In addition, knowing you are loved and protected by the universe also helps you feel less alone. The longer you are single, the more comfortable it becomes because you overcome any fears about being on your own. Then when you are ready, you will meet the person who will truly add to your life.

SELF-ENQUIRY REFLECTION 2.7

....

You may have had an unhappy experience with someone in your past, and this is making you want to be single. However, not letting a bad experience from your past affect your future happiness is an act of courage. These questions will help you become comfortable with enjoying your single life even if you are looking for a partner.

I have the courage to not be in a relationship.

1. On a scale of 0–10 (10 being the maximum), how much do I view being single as a negative experience?

2. What are the benefits of being single compared to being in a relationship?

3. How can I reframe being single into a positive experience?

4. What am I learning about myself from being single at the moment?

5. What action can I take to ensure I enjoy my single life?

LIFE LESSON

....

Do not fear being single. This is an empowered place to be as it means you are less likely to start an unhealthy relationship or be afraid of leaving a relationship. Knowing you can live life on your own, without needing someone around you, teaches you how to be strong and make empowering relationship and life choices.

TOPIC 2.8 HOW DO I KNOW IF I AM
TRULY IN LOVE WITH MY PARTNER?

It can be difficult to know if you are in love with your partner, especially at the start of a relationship due to experiencing a multitude of chemical hormones which can make you feel confused. However, the feelings which are making you think you are in love can be due to the release of oxytocin, the hormone nick-named, *the love drug*. Oxytocin is released when you feel safe, happy and content with someone, yet levels have also been found in people who are in stressful situations. Because of this chemical confusion, it is important to be able to recog-nise loving behaviours demonstrated by your partner, rather than the hormone tricking you into thinking you are in love.

You may not have been taught to identify loving behaviours, therefore these questions will help you identify if you are in a truly loving relationship.

Does your partner:

- embarrass you in private or public and if you challenge them, they tell you that *you are being too sensitive* or *cannot take a joke?*
- show genuine concern for you and help you in hard times?
- stick up for you and protect you when others are being mean to you?
- encourages you to have your own interests and see your friends and family or do they make you feel guilty if you want to do things without them?
- try to understand how you feel, even if they disagree with you and endeav-our to not hurt your feelings?
- give you backhanded compliments which feel insincere?
- want you to do what they want to do and apply pressure when you don't?
- downplay their unacceptable behaviour and not take responsibility for their behaviour, even making you think you are in the wrong when you call out their unacceptable and non-loving behaviour?
- get drunk, mistreat you and then blame the alcohol for their behaviour?
- raise their voice, uses put-downs, sarcasm, sulks, humiliates you or bullies you in anyway?
- play the victim and says manipulative things such as '*I just want to be with you, why don't you want the same'?*

Remember love lifts you up and is not meant to hurt you, while control con-fuses and undermines you, making you question yourself and your worth. Just because your partner tells you they love you, it doesn't mean they do or that you have to respond in the same way. However, if your partner consistently demonstrates loving behaviour, then feel confident in expressing your love.

SELF-ENQUIRY REFLECTION 2.8

· ·

Even in a controlling relationship, there are moments of what appears to be care and consideration shown to you which can be confusing; however, this is not always genuine. These questions will help you discern if your relationship really is loving.

I have the courage to recognise a loving relationship.

1. On a scale of 0–10 (10 being the maximum), how much do I believe I am in a loving relationship?

2. Why do I think my relationship is loving?

You may feel attracted to your partner as they are skilled at making you feel wanted, needed and loved through the words they say. However, do their behaviours and actions make you feel the same way?

3. What loving and unloving behaviours do my partner and I demonstrate towards each other?

4. What percentage of our relationship is joyful, harmonious and loving? What percentage is challenging, argumentative and causing me confusion?

Remember love lifts and empowers while control confuses and belittles. While disagreements are natural in any relationship, resolving them in a caring way is a sign of a loving relationship.

5. What resources can help me learn more about recognising love in a relationship?
   (*internet, friends, family, coach, counsellor, social media, self-help books*)

LIFE LESSON

· · · · · · · · · · · · · · · · ·

Discovering you are in an unloving relationship can be a shock; however, it is better to see the reality of the situation than continue to get hurt. You may have attracted the relationship as you do not feel truly lovable yourself and so learning to love yourself means you then attract genuine loving relationships into your life, and you will have no doubts about expressing your love.

TOPIC 2.9 I AM UNCOMFORTABLE WITH CERTAIN SEXUAL ACTIVITIES

Sexual relationships are a huge learning curve as you learn about your body, your desires and discern what you feel comfortable with. You may feel pressure to lose your virginity or even give in to the sexual demands of another and this can cause you to worry. A consensual relationship is romantic, intimate or sexual in nature, either past or present, to which both parties consent or consented.

The internet has given increased awareness of sexual activity, and because of this, you may be encouraged to take part in activities which you do not want. You may also be comparing yourself to others when you listen to their experiences, or a persistent partner may call you *frigid* or *cold* if you say no to things.

Remember these simple guidelines.

- You should never do anything you do not feel comfortable with.
- No one should bully or manipulate you into anything you don't want to do.
- Someone who cares about you will not bully or manipulate you.

Having sex with someone who has not consented is *assault* or *rape* and is a very serious crime. Consent must always be given, meaning you give the other person permission. If you become uncomfortable, anxious or scared while having sex, you can withdraw consent and if you were intoxicated in any way, you were unable to give your consent, and this is a crime. However, be aware that staying quiet and saying nothing to the other person during the sexual act does not count as consent.

Your partner may say he or she wants you to be adventurous and try other activities such as having a threesome, using sex toys, watching porn, or participating in anal sex. Again, you should not be pressurised into trying anything you do not want to do. If the other person says, '*you would if you loved me*', then this is emotional manipulation and is not authentic love. Remember, sex is a beautiful experience with someone who truly loves and cares for you.

It is an act of empowerment to be in control of your body, go at your own pace and know that you have choices. In a loving relationship, you communicate honestly and openly about trying different sexual activities. If you have felt pressurised to agree to certain activities in the past, forgive yourself for behaving in this way – you maybe didn't realise you felt pressurised into it.

SELF-ENQUIRY REFLECTION 2.9

. . . .

Learning as much as you can about sex and being aware of your own sexuality is part of maturing. You are not wrong or strange for not wanting to partake in sexual activities when you do not feel comfortable. Allowing another person access to your body is not a right, it is something you give permission for.

I have the courage to say no if it makes me feel uncomfortable.

1. On a scale of 0–10 (10 being the maximum), how much pressure am I feeling in sexual relationships?

2. What am I feeling pressurised about?

3. How is the other person pressurising me?

4. How can I communicate I am not happy to proceed?

5. Who can I speak to for further advice about this subject?

   (*community sexual services, counsellor, friend, internet, family, tutor*)

LIFE LESSON

. . . .

Your sex life is your private business, and you can be as open as you wish about the activities you engage with. You may hear other people talk openly about their sexual activity, however being intimate is a loving act and it is okay to go at your own pace and keep your sex life private if you wish to do so.

TOPIC 2.10 MY PARTNER WANTS US TO BE EXCLUSIVE, BUT I DON'T

....

An exclusive relationship is where two people agree that neither of them is romantically pursuing other partners. You may be the person wanting this agreement from the other person, or you may be feeling pressurised by another to upgrade your relationship to this status. Either way, it is important you take the time to reflect on what you really want and not give in to the other person simply for a quiet life or to avoid the relationship ending.

If you are the one who still wants to connect with other people, then exclusivity may make you feel trapped or controlled in some way. Exploring connections with others is your right and is an exciting journey – to settle at a young age is not always the right option for some people. However, sometimes the fear of getting hurt can cause you to avoid committing to a relationship and this fear can prevent you from enjoying a deeper connection with the person who is asking you to be exclusive.

To manoeuvre your way through this situation, it is important to:

- take time to think about what you really want from the relationship;
- not be coerced into behaving in a way that you don't want to;
- communicate how you feel honestly, even if you feel scared;
- do not be afraid of ending the relationship if the status is not what you want;
- let your feelings guide you – do not let fear stop you from following your heart.

You may be the person wanting your partner to be exclusive and he or she is resisting. This can be upsetting for you so be kind and compassionate with yourself. Sometimes it can take time for the other person to realise the depth of their feelings for you and patience is needed before they reach the same level of commitment. However, if it is causing you emotional pain, then explore why exclusivity is so important to you or consider ending the connection. The other person may simply have too many fears to commit to one person. Alternatively, you may have picked a person who is simply not the exclusive type and wants a 'fuck-buddy'. While this can sometimes suit both people, entering this type of relationship when you want a deeper connection can be emotionally challenging. If you want exclusivity, then find someone who feels the same way about you and who doesn't want to risk losing you.

SELF-ENQUIRY REFLECTION 2.10

....

If you and your partner are at different stages in your relationship you may spend time obsessing about them which can affect your mental health. These questions will help you discern what you truly want.

I have the courage to be in a relationship status of my choosing.

1. The type of relationship I want to be in is ...
   (*fuck-buddy, exclusive, boyfriend/girlfriend, friendship*)

2. I want this level of commitment because ...

3. The type of relationship my partner wants is ...
   (*have you asked them why they want the relationship status they want?*)

Most people just want to be loved, nurtured and accepted by another, yet learning how to show this to yourself is important. This is called self-love and the more self-love you have, the more loving relationship you will attract.

4. How much am I compromising what I really want, simply to make the other person happy or because it is more comforting than being alone?

5. How can I create a life where I learn to love, nurture and accept me more?

LIFE LESSON

....

Relationships can cause distress; however, the clearer you are about what you will and won't accept, the happier your relationship experience will be. Being able to walk away from a relationship because you are brave enough to be alone, means you increase the likelihood of having relationships which nurture and fulfil you.

TOPIC 2.11 MY PARTNER HAS POOR MENTAL HEALTH AND I DON'T KNOW HOW TO HELP

Being in a relationship with a partner who struggles with their mental health can be challenging for you both. You may feel you want to take their pain away in some way and this can make you super sensitive to their needs, wants and wishes. Because of this, you may neglect your own needs and find yourself feeling burdened and overwrought with worry about them.

This relationship is called a co-dependent relationship which signifies a degree of unhealthy clinginess and neediness as either one of you is depending on the other for some sort of fulfilment. It is important both parties have the ability to self-soothe and manage their own emotions.

When one partner in a relationship has mental health challenges this can be difficult as self-doubt, a lack of self-trust and fear is present in their life. Their negative outlook is often rooted in adverse childhood experiences where they felt unlovable and were not taught to manage and regulate their own emotions. They therefore rely on another to support them emotionally and mentally. While this can make you feel needed, wanted and validated; the constant support you offer can be draining. Your partner will start to truly heal when they learn how to create a mindset of self-belief, trust in themselves and have a positive outlook.

If your partner feels as though you are withdrawing your support, their behaviour can become obsessive, needy and even manipulative. This is because their deepest fear of abandonment has been activated and they believe they need you to survive. In effect, you may be acting as the nurturing parent, they never had.

Behaviours they may employ if you do withdraw your support.

- Obsessively calling and texting you.
- Crying, shouting, screaming, smashing things, being aggressive – even physically violent.
- Telling you they feel suicidal, or they are going to hurt themselves and it will be your fault.
- Intimating they will 'get worse' if you don't do x, y or z.
- Accusing you of a lack of love if you assert your own needs over theirs.
- Sulking, ghosting you, disappearing or blocking you so you worry or feel guilty.
- Telling you that you have changed, and you don't love them anymore.

The most loving gift you can give to your partner is to not accept this behaviour and encourage them to heal this inner pain through seeking professional help so they can learn to be self-sufficient. This then means your relationship will be one of balance and harmony, where you can both support each other. Alternatively, they may choose to reject support and you may therefore decide to end the partnership as you realise you deserve someone who will support you as much as you support them. You may also want to explore why you existed in such a relationship as it can indicate unmet childhood needs on your part which need to be healed.

SELF-ENQUIRY REFLECTION 2.11

You may be in a co-dependent relationship without even realising, driven subconsciously to fix, support, rescue and heal your partner in some way. Alternatively, you may think you can only be happy if you have someone in your life. These questions will help you discern if you are in a co-dependent relationship.

I have the courage to prioritise my own mental health.

1. Out of 100 per cent, what percentage does my partner support, encourage and nurture me and what percentage do I do this for them?

2. What have I realised about myself, my partner and my relationship from answering question 1?

3. What does my partner offer me – what may you be co-dependent on them for?

4. How do I think my partner and I need to change to make our relationship better? (*you or your partner may need professional help or utilise self-help resources to help you both become more independent*)

Remember you cannot change another person – a person can only take responsibility to change themselves. If you do not see another person taking action to change themselves, you may have to walk away for your own sanity.

5. Where can I learn more about co-dependent relationships? (*internet, self-help books, counsellor, social media*)

LIFE LESSON

Being responsible for your own mental health means you continually reflect on what you are thinking and how you are feeling as situations in your life may be causing you pain. When you do this, you will know the empowering choices you have to make in your life.

TOPIC 2.12 I DON'T KNOW HOW TO SAY NO TO DEMANDS AND REQUESTS FROM OTHERS

Overcoming the internal turmoil caused by saying no to a demand or request from another is essential for your well-being. If you find yourself saying yes when you really want to say no, then you can feel resentment and anger towards the other person and yourself. Saying no to another can often mean you are saying yes to yourself.

However, you may struggle to say no due to avoiding consequences such as:

- hurting the person's feelings;
- being not liked by the person (rejection);
- being criticised and disapproved of;
- disappointing them;
- facing possible conflict and confrontation.

Saying no is one way of demonstrating assertive behaviour. Being assertive is essential in life as there will be some situations where saying no is needed to avoid overwhelm and burnout. You will find an abundance of material on the internet to help you learn more about the valuable subject of assertive behaviour.

Saying no is an example of setting a boundary, making clear what you are willing to tolerate and not tolerate from another person. This is great for your well-being as it means you choose to behave in ways which bring you joy, rather than being coerced into doing something through duty, guilt or control.

Of course, you need to communicate your boundaries, and it is understandable you may feel apprehensive. However, once you realise you have a right to do this, you will appreciate it as a way of taking responsibility for your well-being.

Having a strong sense of self and high levels of self-belief means you have the confidence to set boundaries and do not fear another's reactions. Some people confuse assertion with aggression, but they are not the same. Assertive behaviour does not belittle or wound the other person, whereas aggressive behaviour is rooted in fear, intimidation and control and can leave the other person feeling helpless.

Once you find the courage to set a boundary, the other person may not like this and might call you selfish or say you don't care about them. This may cause you to feel guilty, meaning you concede to the other person. However, remember you always have a right to set a boundary and stand up for yourself – it is a form of self-protection and is an act of self-love.

SELF-ENQUIRY REFLECTION 2.12

....

Boundaries are useful to stop behaviours which you are no longer willing to tolerate from another. These questions will help you understand more about the type of boundaries you would like to think about setting.

I have the courage to set boundaries.

1. What or who is causing me anger, upset, frustration or any other negative thoughts and feelings?

2. If I had a magic wand, how would I want this situation to be improved?

3. Does the improved situation mean I have to change my behaviour, or the other person must change their behaviour? (*the answer will help you discern if it is a boundary for you or the other person or both*)

Remember you do not have the power to change another's behaviour, all you can do is disclose with them what you are no longer willing to tolerate. Only they can then choose to change this behaviour. If they don't, you may need to re-think your connection with them.

4. What fears may be stopping me from setting a boundary with the other person and how can I learn to overcome these fears?

5. How can I learn more about setting boundaries including saying no to others? (*internet, self-help books, coaching, counsellor, tutor, parent*)

LIFE LESSON

....

Learning how to set boundaries will help you achieve your potential, both personally and professionally. The more you learn to set boundaries, the easier it becomes. A person willing to communicate their boundaries is an assertive person.

TOPIC 2.13 I AM CONFUSED ABOUT MY GENDER IDENTITY

....

Over the past few years, society has become more accepting of differences in gender identity. You may have a strong sense of not fitting with the gender you were assigned at birth. Because of the social pressure to behave in a certain way and fear of those around you not accepting or understanding how you are feeling, you may have kept your thoughts and feelings to yourself. Understandably this can make you feel unhappy, lonely or isolated from those around you meaning your mental health suffers.

Accepting and embracing how you think and feel is an important part of loving and respecting yourself. When you do not feel part of a tribe, you can question what is wrong with you; however, there is nothing wrong with you.

Gender identity can be a complex issue. For example, you may feel you can't identify with being either male or female or that you feel you are both male and female or even that you have been in the wrong body since early childhood. Gender identity isn't related to sexual orientation in any way, and you may identify as straight, gay, lesbian, polysexual, pansexual or asexual while being binary, non-binary or transgender. Sexuality and gender identity can also be fluid; that is, they change over time.

You may fear talking to your family or friends about your gender identity, but it is important you find someone who can listen and support you.

Your gender identity is about understanding:

- who you are;
- how you see yourself;
- what people expect of you.

It can take time to learn this, however, exploring the subject now means you can become more comfortable being the person you want to be. Many older people feel they must conform to what their family and society expect of them and therefore struggle all their life not acknowledging their true gender identity.

Find the courage to explore this topic with someone who will be accepting of how you feel and the challenges you are facing. Those who really love you will want you to be happy and you may be surprised at how supportive they are. It is true some family members may not be as understanding as you would like, but this is usually based on how they were raised and what they were taught to believe is right and wrong. Even if your family or those around you do not support you in your decision, there will be someone who will show you the respect and support you deserve.

SELF-ENQUIRY REFLECTION 2.13

. . . .

Having the courage to question and explore your gender identity can help you feel happier and less confused. Being able to reflect and explore your gender is an act of self-respect. Those who unconditionally love you will want you to be happy.

I have the courage to choose my own gender identity.

1. On a scale of 0–10 (10 being the maximum), how confused do I feel about my gender identity?

2. What am I confused about?

3. How does admitting my confusion make me feel?

4. What support do I need which will help me be less confused or help me explore this subject further?

5. Who can I turn to for more support?
   (*friends, family members, internet, support groups, personal tutor*)

LIFE LESSON

. . . .

Being comfortable with every aspect of who you are is an important act of self-love and having the courage to be different to the majority is important. Whatever you are experiencing there will always be someone, even a stranger who has been through a similar experience and wants to support you.

TOPIC 2.14 I THINK I HAVE A FRENEMY IN MY FRIENDSHIP GROUP

Friends can have an amazingly positive impact on your life as they can support you, make you laugh, stop you from doing stupid things, help you process unhappy feelings and encourage you to do well. Quality over quantity is important and just a couple of close friends can be more beneficial than having many shallow friendships, including fake social media friends.

Just like any relationship, friendships can develop and evolve, or you can grow apart, so much so that you may want to let go. This is natural and you don't have to keep the same people in your life forever. However, sometimes it is reassuring to have a group of friends with whom you share old memories; you may just choose not to see them as often as your new friends.

Some friendships are not good for you and can be toxic to your mental health. You may refer to this person as a *frenemy* – someone who may be friendly to you despite a dislike or rivalry.

A frenemy can behave in some of the following ways.

- They only talk about their problems as their emotional needs outweigh yours.
- They do not seem happy about your achievements.
- They talk down or belittle you or even talk about you behind your back.
- They can make cruel comments but see it as being supportive in some way.
- They ask for constant favours and rarely offer you time, support or help.
- They are hypersensitive and you fear upsetting them.
- They are very opinionated about how you live your life.
- They can be jealous if you spend time with other friends.
- They may say horrible things about other friends behind their backs.

You know if you have a frenemy as you feel you cannot be your authentic self with them, somehow guarding what you share with them. This can be tiring and stressful as you are being fake. You may want to resolve this situation by expressing how you feel to this person. Their behaviour may not change but you may feel better for sharing your truth. If you feel you cannot share your truth, then you may need to consider ending the friendship or simply distancing yourself from this person.

You deserve to have friends around you who love and support you, wanting you to be the best version of yourself. They don't always have to agree with you, but you can have open and honest conversations, resulting in a shared respect.

SELF-ENQUIRY REFLECTION 2.14

. . . .

Finding friendships which nurture and support you is important for your well-being. These questions will help you reflect on the friends you have in your life enabling you to discern if they are good to have around.

I have the courage to let go of those who do not nurture my soul.

1. On a scale of 0–10 (10 being the maximum), how concerned am I that I may have a frenemy in my friendship group?

2. Why do I believe this?

3. How do I feel when my friend behaves in this way?

4. What choices do I have to resolve this situation?

5. What resources can help me in learning more about this subject?
   (*internet, social media, self-help books, tutor, coach, counsellor, parent*)

LIFE LESSON

. . . .

Being able to choose good friends is a great skill to have. Friends need to be on your team, not make life harder for you. Letting go of people who do not nurture your soul is great for your mental health and future happiness.

CHAPTER 3
MANAGING FAMILY DYNAMICS

....

Blood makes you related. Love and loyalty makes you family.

Author unknown

SCENARIO

....

Li put her phone down, close to tears after face timing with her family. She loved them dearly but was feeling increasingly despondent each time she spoke with them. Li looked across the room and sighed as she watched her friends Lucinda and Ami in fits of giggles as they stalked Ami's new love interest on Instagram. She loved the friends she had met at university but also felt quite envious of them; they seemed so carefree and happy, whereas Li rarely did. She felt a constant pressure in her head from the moment she woke to the minute she went to bed. She had confided in Lucinda and Ami about the sense of overwhelm she constantly felt, and they had commiserated with her, yet Li knew they didn't really understand the pressure to perform that she consistently felt.

For as long as she could remember Li had put herself on a pedestal, constantly demanding perfection of herself, pushing herself to achieve the best grades possible. However recently she had started feeling panicky, out of breath sometimes, and a sense of doom would descend over her, so much so she had taken to staying in her room to try and help herself feel better. Not wanting to worry her parents, she kept quiet about how she felt when they spoke as she knew they wouldn't understand. Li spoke to them every Saturday evening without fail as they didn't like it if she was unable to take their call.

Li knew her parents were proud of her as they told her constantly, but she wished they wouldn't as it just added more pressure to how she was already feeling. She felt she was dropping the ball in every area of her life, but failure was not an option for Li as the shame of failing would be too much to bear. Lucinda and Ami had tried to encourage Li to go easy on herself, to take the pressure off having to achieve top marks and to not let her family drain her so much, but Li didn't believe this was right, let alone know how to achieve this.

Her older brother had dropped out of medical school two years ago to go travelling and she had witnessed the pain and disappointment it had caused her family. They had taken it personally as though they, the parents, had failed in some way, simply because her brother wanted to experience the world and re-think their plan of him becoming a doctor.

Li loved her family immensely and was grateful they had supported her throughout her life, but sometimes the feelings of having to achieve and be *someone* who they wanted her to be felt too much of a burden. Sometimes Li felt like she wanted to run away, escape from the world she lived in, leaving everything behind. She was having a recurring dream that her family were running after her as she ran naked along the beach, eventually she dived headfirst into the sea, swimming underwater as they called her name. She would wake up with a start, sweating profusely, and it was with a heavy heart that she would realise she was back in reality, one of pressure, responsibility and a nagging feeling of not being good enough.

Remember ... you've got this

Part of the university experience is learning to manage your family's expectations. Being independent means acting in a way where you are free from outside control, not subject to another's authority and able to make your own life choices. Yet this can take time, courage, practice and patience.

Not only are you learning how to become independent, but your family is going through their own transition period, letting go of having responsibility for you. Of course, this is a process and like any journey can have its ups and downs. Letting go and seeing someone deal with the consequence of being responsible for their life choices can be hard and therefore some families struggle to do so.

MANAGING FAMILY DYNAMICS

You are at an age now where you can make your own decisions, and this often means making your own mistakes. However, in reality, there is no such thing as a mistake, as everything which happens to you in your life is a learning experience, giving you valuable knowledge and insights into how to live your life, as long as you learn the soul lessons of course.

Moving from being dependent on another to independent often requires the setting of boundaries. These are like agreements which determine the behaviour you will tolerate or not. Of course, some people don't like you setting boundaries as it means they lose control, which can then trigger their fear making them angry and more controlling, often resorting to threats of what they will do if you fail to do as they say. Yet know you have a right to set boundaries with another, whoever they are. Li may need to set some boundaries with her parents if she wants to become more independent. Perhaps FaceTiming her parents every Friday night is not what Li wants but she is maybe complying from a place of duty, obligation and guilt. However this can cause feelings of resentment, anger and bitterness which is unhealthy for the human body and mind.

Honest conversations are important when relationship dynamics are changing and being open and transparent with those you love will ensure the love and respect remains. Sometimes honest conversations can be upsetting, especially if the other person gets angry or withdraws from you. However, knowing you have a right to speak your truth, means you act with dignity, integrity and courage. If Li can tell her parents how she truly feels, then some of the stress and pressure she is experiencing will reduce.

Reaching out to to tell another how you are feeling is essential when you are feeling stressed or unhappy. It is understandable to feel this way when you are trying to deal with too much on your own. If Li can understand that the pressure she is putting herself under is too much and learn ways to be kinder to herself and know it is okay to fail in life, then her mental health will improve.

Fail can stand for first attempt at learning, and when you are learning a new subject, it is understandable that you will fail sometimes. Not being afraid of failure while at university and throughout your life is essential for personal and professional success.

Li's family may not be as disappointed in her as she thinks, and even if they are, at least Li will know she spoke her truth and can find other people who won't shame Li for feeling the way she does but want to help her relive the stress and pressure.

TOPIC 3.1 MY MENTAL HEALTH IS POOR, BUT I DON'T WANT TO TELL MY FAMILY

Attending university can seem challenging because you are faced with many different external pressures which you may not have encountered before such as:

- learning how to study independently;
- working – either paid or voluntary;
- managing new relationships including existing relationship dynamics;
- balancing social activities;
- learning to live on your own, without others' support.

Your new environment can ask a lot of you, and it is understandable you may start to feel overburdened which can then affect your mental health. Sometimes too many new experiences are being demanded of you, but learning how to balance these demands and admitting how you really feel and asking for help, are all part of your new university experience.

You may think you are weak for feeling overwhelmed, and because of this, you may not want your family to know you are struggling with your mental health as you may not want to worry them. However, if you are struggling, this simply means that your thoughts, feelings and behaviour need to change in some way. It doesn't mean you have something biologically wrong with you, simply that you need guidance and support to deal with the demanding environment you are in.

Even though the role of a parent is one of guidance, nurture and support, they may feel confused about how to help you in this situation, especially if they struggle with their own mental health. Parents are humans themselves and can be unsure of the best way to help you, especially if they have not experienced university. You may be used to automatically reaching out to them for support but on this subject, they may not know the best advice to give. Ask yourself, what response would be the most helpful from them to you at this time and try to communicate this to them.

You may like them to:

- reassure you that you will handle whatever is happening to you;
- acknowledge how hard this is for you and how proud they are of you;
- encourage you to seek support from someone at university;
- ask you what you need from them right now;
- give you a practical piece of advice on how to resolve a certain situation.

Being able to ask your family for what you need is a sign of assertiveness and can help alleviate the pressure they may feel to help you.

Some of you may not have your parents active in your life or, because of their own struggles, they are unable to support you and if this is true for you it is important you seek help from another source. It may also be that your culture may have social norms which prevent you from admitting you are struggling emotionally and therefore you may feel unable to do this. However, the nature of being human can be one of suffering at times and being able to seek the right guidance from the right person will help ease this suffering.

SELF-ENQUIRY REFLECTION 3.1

....

Being open and honest about how you are truly feeling is important for your well-being. Asking for help is a great skill to possess and it is certainly not weak to admit how you are really feeling. These questions will help you understand what your fears are in talking to others about how you currently feel.

I have the courage to admit how I am really feeling.

1. On a scale of 0–10, (10 being the maximum) how worried am I about my mental health?

2. What is preventing me from talking to my family or others about how I feel?

3. What evidence do I have they will react in this way?

4. How would I like them to react and how can I explain what I need from them?

5. Who else can I reach out to for support?
   (tutor, extended family member, friend, counsellor, coach, support group)

LIFE LESSON

....

Your environment can create pressures which challenge your mental health and make you feel unhappy. If you can be mindful of the different pressures, you are facing then this will help you identify action you can take to reduce your overwhelm. Throughout life, you can seek higher wisdom from those who have the correct training, skills and knowledge to help you.

TOPIC 3.2 MY FAMILY ARE CRITICAL OF MY ACADEMIC PERFORMANCE

To receive approval and validation from your family for your academic performance is wonderful but when this doesn't happen it can hurt you emotionally. You may be pleased with your results as you know how hard you have worked; however, your family may be critical or judgemental because your results are not what they expected.

Alternatively, you may not have achieved the results you wanted and reached out to your family for some commiseration. When this is not forthcoming from them, it can make you doubt yourself and your abilities. This lack of support can result in you thinking you are not clever enough to study at university. However, consider the following.

1. It may be that your family hasn't attended university and therefore do not appreciate how different the higher education learning process is from the way you were taught at school and college. This lack of awareness can make them insensitive to how challenging this learning transition is for you.
2. The grading system can be complex to those who are not used to it and your family may expect you to obtain top marks, not fully understanding how unrealistic this can be.
3. Perhaps your family has forgotten that not only are you learning how to be responsible for your academic studies, but you are also exploring how to be independent in every other area of your life, such as cooking, shopping, laundry, diet, financial management, working and maintaining your well-being. This all needs to be commended, as learning to balance all these extra demands takes time, energy and resilience.
4. Some family members expect their child to excel in every way which can put pressure on you to consistently perform. However, it is not your job to be a perfectionist in everything you do (there is no such thing) and remembering this throughout your university experience will help you effectively manage the demands and pressures being placed upon you.
5. Some family members can struggle to compliment, encourage, validate and praise their children, perhaps if they were not supported in this way themselves. They may view their criticism as constructive, pushing you to perform better, however in reality the opposite can happen, or you suffer from burnout trying to achieve unreasonable expectations.

There can be many reasons why your family may be critical of your performance; however, the only opinions which truly matter are yours and your tutors'. If you want accurate, honest feedback, both complimentary and constructive, then reach out and arrange a meeting with your tutor to discuss your current performance.

SELF-ENQUIRY REFLECTION 3.2

....

Other people's reactions, especially members of your family can trigger your insecurities. Not allowing another to have this power over you is essential for your well-being. These questions will help you understand how you can manage this situation better, resulting in improved communication.

I have the courage to seek positive and constructive feedback.

1. On a scale of 0–10, (10 being the maximum), how critical are my family of my academic performance?

2. If they are not critical, what can I tell myself to help me feel better?

3. What feedback do I expect from my family and, what do I receive?

Many older adults seek the approval of their family, but may never receive this, which leaves them feeling disappointed and resentful. It is therefore important to learn how to approve, love and validate yourself and find support from others who you respect.

4. Who can I turn to for the feedback and encouragement I desire? (*tutor, academic staff, friends, other students, internal message boards, counsellor, partner*)

5. What can I say to myself to help approve, love and validate myself?

LIFE LESSON

....

Being your own cheerleader is important; however, there will be times when you will need and want another to encourage and support you. Recognising who can do this for you is important. Sometimes the people who you expect it to be are simply not capable, resulting in disappointment. Ensure you surround yourself with those who want you to succeed, even if this is not your family.

TOPIC 3.3 I CAN'T TELL MY FAMILY I AM FAILING AS THEY WILL BE DISAPPOINTED IN ME

University can be much more challenging than you thought, and it is not uncommon to fall behind in your studies. You may also be struggling emotionally, feeling as though you are drowning, clueless about how you are going to catch up. This can result in you feeling overwhelmed, questioning your competence and as a result, you may stay quiet, in denial about how overwhelming the situation is.

You have two choices to help you resolve the situation, you can either *quit* or *commit* and it is important to choose one of these options as if you chose neither, you are stuck, doing nothing to resolve the situation.

Commit means you commit 100 per cent of your time, energy and resilience to resolve this. If you are behind in your studies, ask yourself what action do I need to take to catch up. You may decide to:

1. make a list of how far behind you really are to get the problem in perspective;
2. ask someone to help you prioritise your tasks so you can tackle the most important or urgent ones first;
3. arrange a meeting with your tutor/lecturer to ask for help;
4. identify how you became so far behind – which of your behaviours do you need to own and how can you stop it from happening again?

These are examples of committing and taking proactive steps to resolve the issue. Once you have done this, you can feel proud as you explain the situation to your family. However, some families, on hearing what has happened, may be fearful that you cannot handle university, and may become angry with you for falling behind. However, this anger is their fear and belongs to them, and it is not your job to soothe them. You can reassure them that you have taken steps not only to resolve the issue but have also learned from the experience, but you do not need to take their anger off them.

Quit means you courageously decide that university life is not right for you as you are not enjoying it. You may have realised that you are trying to persevere because you fear your family's reactions if you admit you want to leave. However, being able to make your own choices is an act of maturity regardless of whether others in your life approve. University is not for everybody, and this is okay, just ensure you are not leaving because you think you cannot achieve – speak to your tutor first to see if they agree with your perception.

Be kind to yourself. Falling behind at university is all part of the learning process and berating yourself is not going to help you catch up. With 100 per cent commitment and the right support, you will soon be back on track.

SELF-ENQUIRY REFLECTION 3.3

. . . .

It can feel overwhelming when you fall behind but the key to recovery is facing your reality. Knowing how far you are behind will help you know the steps you need to take to resolve the situation. These questions will help you to take back control.

I have the courage to resolve the situation.

1. On a scale of 0–10 (10 being the maximum) how far behind am I?

2. How have I fallen behind?

It is important to identify if you have fallen behind due to not being interested in the subject which may indicate the degree course you have chosen is not suitable, or if you are simply taking time to transition into a more independent way of learning.

3. What steps can I take to recover from this situation?

4. What help do I need from another to help me recover from this situation and who may this person be? (*tutor, friend, parent, mentor, coach*)

5. How can I ensure I do not fall behind again?

LIFE LESSON

. . . .

Facing your reality takes courage and it is easy to avoid facing a challenging situation. However, resilience develops from facing difficult situations and taking action steps to change the situation. This is true confidence as you are then devoid of any fearful thoughts and anxious feelings because you know your inner-strength helps you deal with anything which comes your way.

TOPIC 3.4 MY FAMILY AND FRIENDS DON'T AGREE WITH SOME OF MY LIFE CHOICES

Moving away to university means you can make more of your own life choices, free from the rules and expectations of others. Exploring who you are as a person, learning to make your own decisions and dealing with the consequences can be both exhilarating and scary at the same time. Occasionally your family and friends may not agree with some of your decisions, for example:

- the amount of effort you are committing to your studies;
- how you spend your free time while at university;
- your sexuality and gender identity;
- how often you stay in contact and visit home;
- your relationship and friendship choices;
- a theology, religion, hobby or interest you take up.

Sadly, some parents feel threatened if their children make different life choices from them, especially if these life choices are not perceived to be traditional or what they perceive as normal. Of course, there is no such thing as normal, and you have a right to reject this way of thinking and behaving. You have a right to create your own traditions.

Part of transitioning into an adult is being able to converse with your parents in an open and honest way, standing up for what you believe is right for you. Of course, this can result in arguments and disagreements which can be upsetting. However, it is important to bear in mind that some parents want you to be happy and their concerns are simply due to them worrying that you are not making choices which will make you happy. Sometimes you and your family may have to agree to disagree which means accepting each other's point of view. Your family views the situation in one way, and you view it differently and this is okay.

Sometimes families may struggle to accept their adult children's life choices and give an ultimatum: 'change your life or leave my life'. This can be extremely painful, even though it can be simply an unwillingness on their part to let go of their perception of the situation.

Occasionally you may have to step away from those who do not have your best interests at heart, no matter what role they have played in your life. Trust that you have a right to be authentically yourself and follow your heart. Take time to find a like-minded tribe who become your soul family, helping you accept the life choices which are right for you.

SELF-ENQUIRY REFLECTION 3.4

....

Learning to make and own your life choices is important so that you are not scared to be the person you want to be. If others disagree with your choices, it may mean they are unable to change the way they view the world. Yet what is important is that you love the life choices you are making and find people who support you unconditionally.

I have the courage to make life choices which are right for me.

1. What life choices do my family disagree with?

2. How does this make me feel?

3. Often uncomfortable feelings are triggered within you if you are not 100 per cent comfortable with your life choices. On a scale of 0–10 (10 being the maximum) how comfortable am I with my life choices?

4. If I have scored under 7, how can I become more comfortable with my life choices? For example, who or what can I reach out to for support?

5. How can my family and I reach a place of acceptance about each other's views?

LIFE LESSON

....

It is an act of self-love to let go of those who refuse to be polite about your life choices, especially if they continue to shame and humiliate you. If you can feel compassion for all involved, especially with those who refuse to see the world differently, then you will find peace in your heart, yet you still don't have to be surrounded by them physically.

TOPIC 3.5 I DON'T KNOW HOW TO MANAGE MY NEEDY/CONTROLLING FAMILY

Whether you are living at home or have moved away, attending university can certainly change the dynamics between you and your family. University is asking you to become independent and think for yourself in all areas of your life which is a big transition to make. However, your family may be used to you being dependent on them and your independence may cause disharmony. Some families adapt well to this time of change, relishing that they are not needed so much, while others struggle to accept a newly independent adolescent and suffer 'empty nest syndrome'.

However, this is not your responsibility to manage, and it is up to your family to seek help to manage this time of transition. Yet being mindful of how challenging this is for all concerned can help relationships remain positive.

Your family may be exhibiting what you term as needy behaviour, expecting you to be in contact with them constantly, requesting to visit or wanting you to come home, especially at holiday times. Yet you may not want to do this as you may have other plans such as being with your new friendship group. Acknowledging your family may be missing you and wanting to be with you is often all that is needed to soothe their demands. Finding a balance between meeting your needs and theirs is important.

This situation can be easily managed with:

- an understanding and appreciation of both parties' needs and wants;
- honest communication between you;
- implementation of boundaries on both sides;
- sticking to and reinforcing these boundaries.

To identify a boundary, firstly determine what the ideal scenario is for you. Then have honest communication to discover your family's expectations. Decide if you can meet their expectations or not and consider compromise if need be. For example, your family may say they want you to ring home every Friday evening, but you feel this is too much. Finding an element of compromise such as texting once a week may make both parties happy. This then becomes your boundary (an agreement between you both). However, sometimes one party may try to override this boundary and make more contact than agreed so it is important to remind them of the agreement you have previously made.

If your family are extremely needy, their behaviour may verge on controlling which is where they emotionally manipulate you into doing something which can make you feel guilty if you don't do what they want. Sadly, emotional manipulation is quite common in families; however, once you recognise it for what it is, you do not need to respond to it. You need super strong boundaries to deal with emotional manipulation however the more you implement your boundaries, the easier managing these situations will become.

SELF-ENQUIRY REFLECTION 3.5

....

Being able to assert your needs with your family is your right. Regardless of how your family may react, you have a right to make choices which are right for you. These questions will help you reflect on what boundaries you need to manage the current situation.

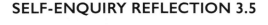

I have the courage to set boundaries with my family.

1. On a scale of 0–10 (10 being the maximum), how needy and/or controlling do I think my family are?

2. How does their behaviour make me think this?

3. What boundaries do I need to implement to reduce the resentment I am feeling?

4. How can I communicate my boundaries in a loving way?

5. What other sources of support can help me manage my family's demands? (*Tutor, counsellor, coach, self-help books, internet, friend, extended family member, mentor*)

LIFE LESSON

....

Transitioning from an adolescent to an independent adult is a process which both you and your family can learn to manage. Being mindful of how this transition is affecting yourself and others will help you become a more compassionate person, benefiting all in the process.

TOPIC 3.6 MY FAMILY DON'T SEEM TO CARE ABOUT ME AS I DON'T HEAR FROM THEM

··

You may feel distanced from your family because you are not seeing them as much, yet out of sight doesn't necessarily mean you are out of their mind. It is understandable you will miss the contact from home, and you may think that you are no longer a priority to your family which can feel scary. You also may have moments of craving to hear from your family but equally become irritated when they try to contact you.

These conflicting emotions are all part of transitioning from being a teenager into an independent adult. Acknowledge it is okay for you to feel confused sometimes and trust that, in time, an equilibrium will be found as you all adjust to the new dynamics.

Some family members may now dedicate their time and energy to their own life, feeling that they have 'done their job' as you have flown the nest. This may leave you feeling unloved or neglected in some way. To resolve this situation, honest, assertive and truthful communication is needed. Having the courage to admit how you feel is key in this situation, after all, how can someone be there for you, if you don't tell them what you need? Maturity is asking the other person how they are feeling about the current situation and being able to hear the answer. Your family may be confused with how they are feeling about you being at university and confused to know how to handle the situation. They may be leaving you alone as they think this is what you want or need. An honest conversation about how you are feeling and what you both need should soon resolve the confusion which has arisen between you both.

Sometimes family members are severely neglectful and have been for all your life, failing to meet your needs, whether those are emotional, mental or physical needs. There is a saying: 'hurt people hurt people'. This means that because of the lack of love they were shown as a child, they never felt loved themselves and are hurting inside, struggling to show you love and care but sadly hurting you in the process.

Of course, not all people who have had a loveless upbringing behave in this way, yet if you are from a family who have neglected you it is important to have compassion for yourself and believe you are lovable, even if it was not mirrored to you. Talking about how you feel with a professional can help you let go of any resentment or sadness you may feel if this has been your experience. In addition, feel proud of how much you have achieved academically without the best start in life and know you have a high amount of inner-strength which has enabled you to get where you are today. This resilience will help you to achieve both personally and professionally in the future.

SELF-ENQUIRY REFLECTION 3.6

....

While it is affirming to receive love and care from another, the most empowering behaviour you can demonstrate is showing yourself love, care and compassion. To love yourself unconditionally allows you to love others in the same way. These questions will help you identify what you are seeking from others and how you can give this to yourself.

I have the courage to show care and love for myself.

1. What behaviour is making me think my family does not care about me?

2. How would I like my family to behave?

3. How have I communicated how I feel to them?

4. How has my past helped me be the resilient person I am today?

5. How can I learn to give this to myself?

LIFE LESSON

....

When you feel insecure and scared, it is understandable you want to reach out to another to help you feel better. However, if you constantly look to another for reassurance without being able to do it for yourself, you can become co-dependent on them, Life is a balance of receiving support yet knowing you have the resilience to survive challenging times.

TOPIC 3.7 | I CONSTANTLY ARGUE WITH MY FAMILY, AND IT DRAINS ME

Arguing with your family can leave you feeling angry, upset, alone, unloved and isolated, especially if they say hurtful things to you. Thankfully some parents, after they have argued with their children are able to apologise, realising they were out of order and will ask you how they can rectify the situation either by compromise or by being willing to accept an alternative point of view. They understand they need to own their part in the disagreement and change their behaviour.

Unfortunately, some parents are unable to do this, perhaps because they did not have this form of compromise modelled to them when they were younger. Therefore, arguments will constantly occur when there is a difference in your beliefs. This means what they think and believe to be true, or right is different to what you think and believe to be true or right. Each person has their own unique way of viewing a situation based on the way they have been raised and sometimes this difference in belief systems means you clash.

If you are drained by constant arguments, seek to:

- understand why your parent believes what they think to be true about the situation;
- explore why you believe your way of seeing the situation is true;
- challenge yourself to see the situation from their viewpoint;
- challenge them to see the situation from your viewpoint;
- ask how you can reach a compromise in this situation.

Remember your family is of a different generation from you and some things in today's world are so different, they struggle to adapt their thinking. They will have a different understanding of the world and disagreeing is okay, it may not mean they love you any less.

However, when someone has believed something to be true for a long time, they can struggle to change their mind. Distancing yourself for a short time until you can each accept each other's point of view can help in these situations. Sometimes the other party may never be willing to change their point of view and you may have to decide whether you want them in your life. Just because someone is family, doesn't mean to say they have to be in your life.

SELF-ENQUIRY REFLECTION 3.7

....

Maturing into an independent adult means being comfortable owning your opinions while being able to accept the opinions of others. You don't have to agree with another as long as you are both respectful of each other's views. These questions will help you identify why you are clashing with another and how you can resolve the situation.

I have the courage to own my beliefs.

1. What am I arguing with my family about?

2. How does arguing with my family make me feel?

3. Why do we both think we are right about the situation we are arguing about?

4. How are my beliefs different to my parents?

5. How can I find some compromise, agree to disagree or alternatively resolve this situation in order that my mental health benefits?

LIFE LESSON

....

Being able to think autonomously is a great skill to have and your maturity will help you realise you can think differently to others, including your family. Being able to own your beliefs while being open to other people holding different beliefs means you learn to evolve and grow psychologically and spiritually as an independent person.

TOPIC 3.8 I AM WEIGHED DOWN BY
THE PROBLEMS OF MY FAMILY

Even though you are at university, you may be worrying about problems that your family are experiencing at home. Perhaps there is illness in your family or disagreements are occurring at home between those you love. It is understandable you feel concerned, or even helpless, especially if your family are looking to you for support.

However, you have a right to live your own life, and this is achieved by being responsible for yourself and by stopping taking responsibility for others. Seeing those you love upset or angry can trigger uncomfortable feelings within yourself and to avoid feeling this way, you may have learned to people please, wanting to resolve their problems over your own. This means you behave in ways to avoid others becoming angry or upset with you, neglecting your own needs in the meantime. However, this can leave you feeling drained and resentful.

If your family struggle to handle challenges and look to you to solve them, remember it is not your role to do this and although it may feel harsh to stop taking responsibility for others, in the long run it will benefit your mental health. If others are struggling to manage, it is their responsibility to seek support from professionals who can help them.

Saying no to someone does not mean you love them less: in fact, the opposite can be true as it is an act of love to help others realise, they do not need you but are able to solve their own challenges. Saying yes to another through guilt and duty may mean you are saying no to yourself. It is okay to say no to another without feeling guilty. Learn to handle your fears of not being liked, approved of, and even being rejected and you will make choices which although may upset others are right for you.

> Imagine the problems you are worrying about as rocks and witness yourself putting these rocks into a rucksack and carrying them around with you. How heavy do they feel? Now stop and sort the rocks into two piles, a pile of rocks which belong to you (those which are your responsibility to resolve) and a pile of rocks which belong to the other person to resolve? Visualise handing these rocks back to the other person to carry – how light does this now make you feel?

Allowing others to take responsibility for their life is a gift to both yourself and them. Allowing them to make choices and be accountable for their choices helps you let go of the pressure you are feeling. You have a right only to be responsible for yourself (unless you have small children or those who are neurologically unable to do it for themselves of course).

SELF-ENQUIRY REFLECTION 3.8

....

Other people in your life may struggle to take responsibility for their life, meaning they fail to behave in empowering ways. This is often because they do not know how to. These questions will help you discern who is not taking responsibility and how you can allow them to do so.

I have the courage to be responsible for myself.

1. Which people in my life do I feel responsible for sorting out their problems?

2. What do I feel I have to resolve for them? (*what are you worrying about specifically?*)

3. Why do I feel I have to resolve their problems for them and how may I not be the best person to do this?

4. How does it feel giving them back their own rocks to carry?

5. What may they learn by taking responsibility to resolve their own problems?

LIFE LESSON

....

Letting go of the need to psychologically fix, emotionally rescue or make other people's lives better can help you focus on making your own life as good as it can be. When you stop behaving in this way, you realise your worth is not tied to how much you please others, but that you are good enough simply for being you.

CHAPTER 4
ENGAGING POSITIVELY WITH ACADEMIC TEACHING STAFF

....

Education is not the learning of facts but training the mind to think

Albert Einstein

SCENARIO

....

Dr Michaels paused for a moment from the PowerPoint presentation he was delivering and looked around the large lecture hall. It was one of his favourites due to the size and shape of the room and the way the windows allowed just enough of the hazy November sun to shine through. He appreciated the natural, rich acoustics which made his voice sound stronger and much more powerful than he was currently feeling.

He had moved to this university at the start of the academic year and was taking more time to settle in than expected. The internal politics seemed to place so many extra demands on him, much more than his previous role at his last university. To add to his pressures, his wife was struggling with the 300-mile move, especially as she had left a teaching job she loved and so far, had not found a new position. His life was certainly stressful at the moment, but he couldn't allow himself to think about it right now.

He cherished being a higher education lecturer, yet the differences in the students who attended his lectures never ceased to amaze him. From those who were fully present, furiously typing notes on their brand-new laptops, to those who seemed far away, deep in thought or doodling mindlessly on their notepads. And then of course there were those students who made it perfectly clear that they would prefer to be anywhere else but listening to him.

He had learned many years ago not to take his students' behaviour personally and had to remind himself constantly that even if he was making a difference to just one student, then the stress and pressure of being an academic lecturer was worth it. Knowing he had inspired a student to believe in their capabilities, seeing them grow and evolve as a person gave his life meaning. To have an engaged student asking questions, challenging his research, and presenting an alternative view made him feel alive. He understood the transition was hard for many of the students, moving from a spoon-fed secondary school environment to one of independent learning. However, after 25 years of working in higher education, he knew most students did adapt with time, patience and commitment.

He also found great pleasure in being a personal tutor as this gave him the opportunity to support students the best he could. He would constantly reiterate to his tutees that they were on the same team, yet he understood they were apprehensive about admitting their struggles to him. However, in time, most came to realise that he was there to support, not criticise, and they slowly learned to trust him and see him as an ally, focused on helping them achieve personal and professional success.

Knowing he had only five minutes left, Dr Michaels brought his mind back to his presentation and started to summarise the findings of his latest research.

Remember ... you've got this

Engaging positively with academic staff will help your university experience be much more enjoyable, increasing your chances of academic success. Appreciating that teaching staff are there to support you, but also push you to be the best you can be, will help you understand you are both working towards the same goal.

It is their responsibility to give you feedback which at times may be difficult or upsetting to hear, hold you accountable to deadlines and apply healthy pressure to help you develop personally and professionally. Remember that honest and open communication with teaching staff about any insecurities you may have will help you gain reassurance and clarity from them.

Of course, teaching staff are human too and can suffer from stress and pressure as they manage other demands on their time, both personal and professional. Being mindful of this will help you build a respectful and trusting relationship. Equally, academic staff are not surrogate parents or mental health professionals and if you are feeling overwhelmed in your personal life, they may need to refer you to an individual or department who can help you in more specialised ways.

If teaching staff struggle to give you the help you need and you have discussed your frustrations with them and the issue hasn't been resolved, then you have every right to consult a third party within the university to help you resolve the situation.

Learning to have professional adult relationships with teaching staff is all part of the university experience and being able to do this, will help you enormously when you are ready to transition into the world of work where honest and assertive communication is key to success.

TOPIC 4.1 I AM SCARED TO ADMIT I AM STRUGGLING AT UNIVERSITY

Asking for help from another can be difficult at the best of times, but admitting you are struggling to understand the content of your lecture to the person who is teaching you can seem scary. In addition, not understanding the content of your lecture can make you question and doubt yourself and because of this you may think you are:

- not clever enough to study at university;
- you are wasting your time and money studying;
- unsure why you came to university;
- you'd be better off at home, earning money like your friends;
- want to give up and return home.

Fear and doubt can make you think this way, so don't berate yourself for having these thoughts. Seeking clarity and reassurance is a better way to spend your time and you may like to consider reaching out to academic staff for help. However, you may be fearful of doing this due to, being scared of:

- getting told off for not understanding content;
- facing disapproval for seeking help;
- ridicule or embarrassment for not knowing the answers;
- failure at having to ask for help.

Once again, these are common anxieties. However, the role of academic teaching staff is to help you to become an independent, critical thinker allowing you to obtain the best result possible and sometimes this means explaining information to you in different ways.

Academic staff appreciate students who ask for help as it indicates they want to learn, succeed and are interested in the subject. The more you overcome your fears and reach out, the more confidence you will feel in yourself. You will learn your fears have no emotional power over you anymore. In addition, remember you have a right to ask for help as your fees contribute towards the lecturer's salary which means you are paying for his or her time.

The first step is always the hardest, and if you think you will struggle to ask the lecturer face to face for help, then send an email requesting assistance. Be specific about what you are struggling with and what help you need. Perhaps they can answer your query over email, or they may suggest you pop in to see them. Learning to be comfortable when talking to academic staff is all part of maturing and the more you do it, the more you will see the benefits as your relationships strengthen.

SELF-ENQUIRY REFLECTION 4.1

....

It is useful to identify what is scaring you the most, asking for help in general or asking your lecturer for help. Being able to overcome your vulnerability of asking for help will help you succeed and achieve your academic potential.

I have the courage to ask for help.

1. On a scale of 0–10 (10 being the maximum), how scared am I of asking for help from the lecturer?

2. What are my specific fears about approaching the lecturer?

The way to overcome your fear is to do the thing you are scared of as you realise fear is just an illusion.

3. What would be the benefits of approaching the lecturer?

4. What action can I take right now to approach the lecturer for help?

5. What encouraging words can I say to myself to help me approach the lecturer for help?

LIFE LESSON

....

Asking for help is a strength not a weakness and recognising when you need help is an important skill. There will always be someone who has experience of your struggles and wants to help you by sharing their knowledge and wisdom with you. Have the courage to reach out for help whatever challenging situation you are facing.

TOPIC 4.2 I DON'T UNDERSTAND A WORD MY LECTURER IS SAYING

Firstly, the way you learn at university is very different from school or college. You are no longer *spoon-fed* by teachers but expected to work alone (hence the term *independent learner*) by researching the subject, comparing different ideas then delivering your knowledge in alternative ways such as a forum, assignment or presentation. This can seem overwhelming at first as you adjust to new ways of working and demonstrating your learning, so try to not doubt yourself as you learn how to do this.

Lecturers can have different ways of introducing the basics of a topic and if you are struggling to understand the foundations of the topic you may struggle to independently research the subject in more detail. This is why it is important to seek clarity at the beginning of your module.

You may have had occasions at school when you didn't understand what was being taught and your parents may have raised this with your teacher. However, at university, you are responsible for resolving these struggles. Like anything, the more you learn to stand up for yourself, the easier it becomes.

To help overcome your challenge, first identify what exactly it is you are struggling with.

- Is the subject content complicated?
- Is it the communication skills of the lecturer – their tone, pace or language?
- Have they assumed you understand the content, failing to check your knowledge?
- Is the way they present material difficult for you?

It is very easy to think it is your lack of intelligence rather than their delivery which is causing you to not understand. Once you have identified the specific issue you are struggling with, ask yourself:

- how can the lecturer help me understand better?
- how can I help myself to understand better?

The most helpful action you can take is to admit you need some further clarification on the subject matter.

SELF-ENQUIRY REFLECTION 4.2

....

The process of learning can be painful and failing is also part of learning. Yet fail can stand for *first attempt in learning* and therefore tenacity is key. Think of learning to tie your shoelaces or learning to ride a bike: you didn't quit after the first attempt.

I have the courage to resolve my confusion.

1. On a scale of 0–10 (10 being the maximum), how much am I struggling to understand my lectures?

2. Which lectures in particular am I struggling to understand?

3. Why do I think I am struggling to understand this particular subject? (*is it the lecturer, the content or both?*)

4. What do I need to help me understand the lecture/lecturer better?

5. What action do I need to take to resolve this issue?

LIFE LESSON

....

When faced with a new learning experience, you may have times when it can feel too much, and you want to give up. However, continue to take small baby steps towards your goals and you will reach success, realising how brave and tenacious you really are in the process. Do not struggle in silence; reach out for help as there will always be someone willing to help.

TOPIC 4.3 I AM AVOIDING ASKING FOR FEEDBACK FROM MY TUTOR/TEACHING STAFF

....

Feedback can be an amazing gift, yet it can feel painful; after all who wants to hear what you have got wrong or misunderstood? However, the reality of being human is that you are always learning in life, and you will always not know something, and this is okay. Part of the learning process is acknowledging that you will get things wrong sometimes, especially at university as you are learning something new. Yet your tutor and academic staff are mentors who can guide you to understand what you have misunderstood and, more importantly, how you can learn from it in order to achieve success. This is the beauty of feedback.

So where did you learn to be afraid of feedback?

At school, the teaching system grades and compares you constantly which may have made you feel inferior and set up a fear of being criticised. Even your parents or family may have compared you to another and you may have felt that you didn't measure up in some way, leaving you feeling vulnerable and insecure.

Accepting that you are allowed to misunderstand things and viewing feedback as positive, means you can evolve into a more conscious and confident individual who recognises constructive criticism as an important tool in achieving success.

Of course, not all feedback is justified and knowing when to push back and challenge is also important. Feedback should be specific and detailed, giving you evidence of how you can improve next time. For example, simply being told you didn't put enough work into an assignment is not adequate feedback and you should ask for more specific examples to help you understand how you can improve next time.

The more you can be open to feedback, the more you can grow and develop as a person. Remember at your core you are good enough regardless of the feedback you receive. You have the power to view feedback in a positive light – helping you to improve your academic skills. You are at university to learn, and feedback can help you become a better student. Being brave enough to ask for feedback is a skill which will serve you well in your life.

SELF-ENQUIRY REFLECTION 4.3

∙∙∙∙∙∙∙∙∙∙∙∙∙∙∙∙∙∙∙∙∙∙∙∙∙∙∙∙∙∙∙∙∙∙∙∙∙∙∙

Being able to ask for and process feedback is a sign of maturity. Of course, it may be hard to hear the first time you receive it, but if you reframe it as helping you to become a better learner then you will see the value in it.

I have the courage to ask for feedback.

1. On a scale of 0–10 (10 being the maximum), how able am I to ask for feedback?

2. What do I dislike about receiving feedback?

3. How would receiving feedback help me achieve my goals?

4. What would I say to a friend who is upset after receiving feedback? (Then tell yourself this.)

5. How would I like feedback in order that it helps and not hinders me?

LIFE LESSON

∙∙∙∙∙∙∙∙∙∙∙∙∙∙∙∙∙∙∙

Being able to ask for and accept feedback in all areas of your life can help you fulfil the roles you play in life. For example, asking your child, how can I be a better parent or asking your partner how can I be a better partner or even asking your boss how can I be a better employee can give you valuable intel and create improved relationships.

TOPIC 4.4 I AM SCARED TO ASK QUESTIONS IN LECTURES

When learning any new subject, it is essential to ask questions to gain clarification. However, you may be apprehensive about asking questions, fearing:

- looking stupid and feeling embarrassed;
- thinking it is a ridiculous question to ask;
- not wanting other students to laugh at you;
- the lecturer thinking you are unintelligent and criticising you;
- getting tongue-tied or unable to express yourself clearly;
- not understanding the answer, you are given.

These are all common fears to have. However, when faced with fear, you have two choices – either '*face it*' or '*fake it*'. Fake it means failing to admit you are scared of asking a question and therefore do not ask any, but then of course your fear remains.

Facing your fears means finding the courage to ask a question which may involve feeling discomfort and apprehension but ultimately you realise you can handle these feelings and your fear disappears, your confidence builds, your insecurity reduces and you no longer fear asking questions in lectures. You realised you can handle it!

Identifying you are fearful in other areas of your life is part of being self-aware and it is useful to ask yourself the following questions.

- What is the worst that could happen if I push through this fear?
- What is the best that could happen if I push through this fear?
- What will happen if I do nothing to push through this fear?

Reflecting on these answers will help you make the right choice, resulting in high levels of self-worth and self-belief. Fear is one of the biggest obstacles you will encounter in your life but taking responsibility for overcoming your fears is one of the most empowering acts you can do.

Remember you have a right to ask a question and it doesn't mean you are stupid or unintelligent, it simply means you need more clarification to help you process the information. It may be the lecturer has not explained the subject correctly or is assuming prior knowledge or simply their teaching style does not suit you. You may be giving the lecturer some valuable feedback as to how they can improve their teaching style. Finally, asking questions also reassures the lecturer you are interested in the topic.

SELF-ENQUIRY REFLECTION 4.4

....

A person who asks questions can think critically, which is an essential skill in the world of academia, fake news and social media. Having the confidence to assert your voice will help you achieve success, both personally and professionally. These questions will help you identify any fears you may have in asking questions.

I have the courage to ask questions.

1. On a scale of 0–10 (10 being the maximum), how fearful am I of asking a question in a lecture?

2. What negative consequences do I think may happen if I ask a question?

3. What evidence do I have to support my answers to question 2?

4. What can I say to myself, to help you overcome any fears I may have?

5. If you are unable to do this, what other solutions can I think of to help me overcome my fear of asking questions? (Approach lecturer at the end of lecture, email the question, input onto forums, raise hand emoji if online.)

LIFE LESSON

....

Being a person who asks questions is the trait of a leader. Even if you receive a negative response, it does not mean your question was wrong. Honouring yourself by having the courage to seek clarification on any subject is an essential skill to have personally and professionally.

TOPIC 4.5 HOW DO I CREATE POSITIVE RELATIONSHIPS WITH ACADEMIC TEACHING STAFF?

Forming positive relationships with academic teaching staff can help your university experience be a positive one, both personally and professionally. You both share the same goal of academic success so working together to achieve this is essential. Like any relationship, being respectful and understanding each other's needs will help you maintain a good working relationship.

To achieve this, open and honest communication is required between you both. In addition, it is important to remember academic teaching staff have other demands on their time and supporting students is only part of their role. Sometimes due to conflicting demands they too may be under a deadline pressure and are not able to see you right away or provide a quick turnaround time with your query. Different members of staff will have their own ways of teaching, marking and communicating with you and it is helpful to be aware of these. The following guidelines can help develop strong working relationships with academic staff.

Seek clarification and ask questions

If you are confused about what is being asked of you, then seek clarification as soon as possible. If you are unsure what the correct protocol is, then ask questions to avoid any confusion which may impact you both.

Be honest

Be clear about how you are feeling – if you are feeling overwhelmed or confused about something then be honest in admitting your vulnerability. They can only help you if they know what you are struggling with.

Be clear

If you are seeking clarification on a subject, then be specific in what you are asking. If you are communicating via email, keep the content as short, clear and unambiguous as possible, in order that your query can be answered. If it is a longer query, ask for a convenient time to speak to them.

Be compassionate

Your teaching staff are human and can get overworked, tired, irritable and stressed just like you can. Not taking anything personally can help you both in this situation.

Be mindful

Your teaching staff have a home life too and may not be able to answer questions out of hours. Be organised and respectful when communicating with them.

ENGAGING POSITIVELY WITH ACADEMIC TEACHING STAFF

Be authentic

If you are feeling angry or frustrated regarding any aspect of the studying process, then it is okay to communicate this. However, be emotionally aware of how you express your feelings. Be authentic but seek to understand rather than condemn.

Remember, your teaching staff are there to support and guide you, and most of them are on your team, wanting you to succeed. However, you are both responsible for creating a solid, respectful and courteous relationship which means both of you respect each other's needs.

SELF-ENQUIRY REFLECTION 4.5

....

Being able to communicate authentically with teaching staff can improve your studying process. Recognising you are both responsible for the relationship will help you build a respectful one, benefiting you both. These questions will help you identify how you can improve your relationship with the teaching staff.

I have the courage to create a solid working relationship.

1. On a scale of 0–10 (10 being the maximum), how good is my working relationship with the academic staff?

2. What is not working so well regarding my relationship with them?

3. What is working well regarding my relationship with them?

4. How can they and I take responsibility to make the relationship better?

5. How would an improved relationship help me now and in my future career?

LIFE LESSON

....

Being able to create good working relationships with people you meet, both now and post-university will contribute towards personal and professional success. Understanding each other's needs and perspectives leads to harmonious relationships. However, be mindful some people are unable to do this, and harmony is impossible, no matter how much you try.

TOPIC 4.6 I AM CLASHING WITH MY ACADEMIC LECTURER

Occasionally, you may have disagreements with academic teaching staff which result in disharmony. However, it is important your academic success is not sabotaged by communication difficulties and disagreements. Even if someone is older than you, it doesn't mean they will always behave in a mature and adult way, they may struggle to communicate authentically. However, you can be the person who initiates action to resolve any disharmony.

It takes courage to address this kind of situation, but the following suggestions may help.

- Ask to have a private meeting with your lecturer as arguing in front of other students is not constructive. Prepare for the meeting by having specific examples of what you are unhappy with. For example, saying, I feel you are being biased towards me without giving evidence-based examples is unhelpful for both of you.
- See your meeting as a debate and come from a position of being curious about his or her behaviour. Do not seek to be right but seek to understand and be understood. Own that you may not be seeing the full picture and ask, what am I not seeing here?
- Be clear on the outcome you want from the meeting, ask yourself what do I hope to achieve by having this conversation? How will you know if the situation has been resolved well for both of you?
- Own your part in the dynamic – ask 'have I said or behaved in a way which has contributed to this situation'? Then be open to hearing the answer and look for evidence-based examples from them too. This is taking responsibility and is important in life.
- Most teaching staff are on your team, and it may be that you are not seeing the bigger picture. For example, you may have taken their feedback as criticism, but from their perspective, they may be trying to help you develop as they know you can do much better as they can see your potential.

Sometimes you may be unable to resolve the situation and may need to refer the matter to a third party for resolution. Your university will have a complaints procedure, however, trying to resolve the situation informally can save time and pain. Talking to another member of staff about the situation, such as your tutor, student services or pastoral, may be a suitable option initially.

SELF-ENQUIRY REFLECTION 4.6

. . . .

Being able to take responsibility to resolve conflict is an essential skill in life. Disagreements can occur but being able to resolve them is important and each of you have a right to be treated with respect. These questions will help you discern what action you can take to resolve any issues you may be having.

I have the courage to resolve disagreements.

1. On a scale of 0–10 (10 being the maximum) how much am I experiencing disharmony with academic teaching staff?

2. What specific struggles am I experiencing and what evidence do I have this is truly happening?

Sometimes we perceive a situation with no direct evidence. We may just have created a story in our head. Could your way of seeing the situation be biased in any way?

3. What action can I take to resolve the situation?

4. What would be the benefits of resolving this situation?

5. Who else could I talk to who will help me resolve this situation? (*student services, pastoral, a different tutor/lecturer*)

LIFE LESSON

. . . .

You may be fearful about having an honest conversation to resolve this issue; however, the more you learn to do this, the easier it becomes. It is realistic to expect to have disagreements with people in your life and you are not expected to like everyone but communicating honestly and openly in order to obtain your goals is important throughout your life.

CHAPTER 5
MANAGING LECTURES, SEMINARS AND TUTORIALS

Life begins at the end of your comfort zone.

Neale Donald Walsh

SCENARIO

Aisha was struggling both mentally and emotionally – pretending she was fine and had everything under control. Yet, on the inside, Aisha felt as though she was getting sucked into a big black hole, each day feeling increasingly overwhelmed, helpless and confused.

It was week five of her first semester at university and after the excitement of the first few weeks of meeting new friends and exploring the city and campus, she was now feeling worn out, confused and unhappy – the fun seemed to have quickly disappeared from her new student life.

When Aisha had started university, she truly believed she would master the lectures, keep up with coursework and conquer the reading lists. After all, she was a grade A student throughout school and had experienced great relationships with the teaching staff, yet here she didn't seem to be getting the same results and was struggling to connect with academic staff, making her seriously doubt her ability to succeed.

Struggling to keep up with the reading away from lectures was causing Aisha the most concern. She had even started to skip some lectures just to spend time writing up notes from past lectures. She felt as though the world was on her shoulders and she didn't know which way to turn. Her family back home didn't seem too concerned and rarely contacted her to see how she was doing; they always seemed to be busy doing something else. And anyway, even if they did ring, Aisha wouldn't admit she was struggling, after all, who wants to be seen as a failure, especially when Aisha had rarely failed at anything in her life.

The other challenge Aisha was having was understanding the content of one particular class and had started to feel anxious before the class started.

She would sit in the class and make notes but when she tried to write up her notes at home, they made no sense whatsoever. In addition, the structure of the class was group work which made it worse as she was expected to share her thoughts with others, but would sit there fearful of contributing and said nothing, which of course made her feel even more stupid.

As each week ended, Aisha considered dropping out and going home. Yet the shame of this was making her feel even more helpless. She had thought about visiting the doctor for some anti-anxiety medication to try and make herself feel better.

....

Remember ... you've got this

The thoughts and feelings Aisha is experiencing are common to many students in the first semester at university. This is because learning at university is a very different process from the way you learn at school/college and can take some adjustment. However, the great news is that university teaching staff understand this and are on hand to help you make a smooth transition. Being able to reach out for help, share your concerns and be open to advice is an important part of the university experience.

Primarily Aisha is thinking she is failing which is triggering anxious feelings. The physical symptoms triggered by the fear hormones of adrenaline and cortisol are cascading through her body, stopping her logical and rational thought. This then means she can't seek solutions and feels increasingly out of control. She is on a roundabout of fear.

While Aisha should be applauded for realising she needs help to manage her feelings, the answer may not necessarily lie in medication. Medication may calm her and numb how she feels, but it may not help her deal with the core problem of feeling a failure and overwhelmed. Aisha needs to face her fears and ask for help to prioritise her time and seek reassurance she is doing okay. A session with her tutor on how to adjust to the teaching style at university will help her immensely.

Some students berate themselves if they don't get top grades when starting university. They believe that because they obtained high grades in their school and college examinations the same should be true for university. However, the final grades they achieved at school or college were the result of years of practice and preparation and were not achieved within the first few weeks of learning new subjects. Being more realistic and compassionate to oneself in this instance will help improve your university experience.

Being successful is not just about academic success but being confident in the person you are, realising you can handle new experiences with the minimum of self-doubt and fear. And just like Aisha, the more you take action to get help, the more confident you become, truly believing you can achieve great things, both personally and professionally.

TOPIC 5.1 I AM AVOIDING ATTENDING MY LECTURES AND SEMINARS

You will not be the first person to do this, but the university experience is one of being responsible for making behavioural choices. One of these behaviour choices is deciding whether you attend lectures, seminars and tutorials. It is understandable you will have days when you don't want to attend or other priorities demand your time, and this is okay as long as it doesn't become too much of a pattern.

It is important to understand the reason you are missing or avoiding lectures and seminars. If the thought of attending is causing you worry or anxiety in some way, then you need support in overcoming these fears. If you are not enjoying the subject or find it boring, then discussing this with your tutor would be a good idea. However, it is not realistic to enjoy all your subjects.

If the lecture clashes with something else you would rather be doing, this is also understandable. There is nothing more annoying than a lecture scheduled on a Friday at 5pm when you would rather be sat with your friends celebrating the start of the weekend or on the train home. Alternatively, you may be offered a shift at your part-time job and need the money, or family responsibilities may be demanding your time.

However, becoming independent means weighing up the cost versus the benefit when making a choice. Think about the cost of attending the lecture versus the benefit. A good question to ask yourself is, what would be the most empowering choice in this situation? Remember that any choice made from fear is not empowering and should be avoided. Making choices which are going to enhance your future is a responsible way to live.

Taking responsibility for your university experience means making it the best it can be. Remember you are paying for this experience, so it doesn't really matter to anyone else other than yourself if you don't attend lectures. However, if you don't engage with your learning, you are paying for something but not receiving the benefit. You deserve to give yourself the best chance of success.

Whatever reason you are not attending or engaging with your studies, reach out and speak to your tutor/academic adviser. Their role is to support you in having the best experience possible. Ignoring the non-attendance problem means it may get bigger and cause you to worry. Reaching out for help to overcome this challenge acknowledges that you deserve success and recognition for all the hard work it took to be given a university place.

SELF-ENQUIRY REFLECTION 5.1

....

Making the choice to miss lectures is common for a variety of reasons and some of these reasons will be valid for you. These questions will help you realise why you are missing lectures and help you take responsibility to find a solution. If you are missing lectures due to fear, then you need help to overcome this.

I have the courage to ask for help.

1. Why do I think I am avoiding or missing lectures and seminars?

2. How and when did missing lectures and seminars first start?

3. If a miracle happened and I started attending your lectures, what would have changed?

4. Knowing I can take responsibility to attend lectures, what action do I need to take?

5. Who can I speak to who can help me in this situation?

LIFE LESSON

....

It is often easier to avoid taking action, due to fear of what could happen, and many people deny reality rather than deal with it due to a fear of consequences. However, it is important to identify why you are avoiding a situation. and then take action to face it. This is courage in action and will help you become a more confident, resilient and happier individual.

TOPIC 5.2 I FEEL ANXIOUS ABOUT ATTENDING MY LECTURES AND SEMINARS

....

Anxiety is a common word for people to use. The online Oxford dictionary defines anxiety as a '*feeling of worry, nervousness or unease about something with an uncertain outcome*'. Therefore, it is understandable that you may feel worried, nervous, and uneasy about attending lectures as the outcome is uncertain if you haven't experienced them before.

The worry, nervousness and unease that you are experiencing may be caused by a multitude of things. It may be due to the size of the lecture hall and the number of students attending the lecture. It may be due to a fear of being asked to speak in the lecture or participate in group work. You may feel overwhelmed at the speed the lecturer talks or the way you are expected to make your own notes. Whatever the reasons are as to why you feel anxious, it is important to not judge yourself harshly and have compassion for yourself.

Another way to describe anxiety is to say you are scared, and it is okay to feel this way as the university experience is one of huge transformation personally and professionally. New experiences are continually pushing you out of your comfort zone which can make you feel overwhelmed. However, the only way to get rid of your fears is to find the courage to face them, therefore firstly identify what you feel scared about regarding attending lectures and then have a plan to overcome it.

You may need support in knowing how to face your fears as often when you are immersed in the emotion of something, it can be hard to think of a logical answer. Therefore, it may be a good idea to reach out for support to a friend, lecturer or personal tutor to talk about how you can overcome your anxieties surrounding attending lectures. The more you do the things you fear such as attending lectures or asking your lecturer for help, the easier the event becomes as you know the outcome and the anxiety reduces.

In time you will understand that anxiety is akin to fear, and as you become more resilient, you will realise you could handle the situation all along, you just needed practice. It is common to avoid situations when you feel anxious, but this is not a good idea as you will never learn that you are strong enough to face the new experience. Most people, even older adults, feel apprehensive when faced with new situations, and the biological reaction which is called anxiety is simply your body asking you to check you will be safe. It is a survival instinct, hence why facing the new situation with strength and courage will help you realise it is safe and you will see how resilient you really are. Try re-naming your anxiety fear and see how empowering this is – as you can overcome your fears by facing them.

SELF-ENQUIRY REFLECTION 5.2

....

Feeling anxiety at university is a common emotion. As the physical sensations of anxiety are caused by hormones triggered by your fearful thoughts of what may happen, these questions will help you understand what your fearful thoughts are.

I have the courage to overcome my anxiety.

1. What makes me feel anxious about attending lectures or seminars?

Your answer above may be a story you are telling yourself and often, is unlikely to happen. This is because we often only see the negative side of a situation and even if something similar has happened in the past, this doesn't mean it will happen again.

2. In reality, how likely is it these events will happen?

3. If I thought more positively, what is more likely to happen?

4. If you faced your fears of attending, what baby steps can you take to overcome your fear?

5. Who in the university can you reach out to for support who will help you with this?
   (*Tutor, counsellor, lecturer, student services, pastoral, online guides*)

LIFE LESSON

....

If you can call anxiety your fear, this then stops you from feeling disempowered. This is because the real purpose of anxiety (fear) is to help you become psychologically stronger by learning to face and handle situations with an uncertain outcome. The less you are affected by anxiety, the more confident you are, meaning you will create a life which brings you joy, happiness and success.

TOPIC 5.3 I DON'T UNDERSTAND THE CONTENT OF MY LECTURES AND SEMINARS

Some lectures and seminars can be more difficult to understand than others, but don't give up. The most unhelpful action you can take is to stop going to the lectures, thinking 'what's the point?' It can feel overwhelming when you don't understand the content, and this can make you panic as you feel out of control. However, even admitting you are struggling to understand the content is an act of taking responsibility and puts you back in control.

Sometimes lecture content is boring and it is understandable that you may not find every lecture interesting. If you find it boring, you can lose your motivation and want to give up. However, a lack of motivation can also be a result of self-doubt, so have faith in yourself that you can achieve. If it is a lecture you are not interested in, then trust that eventually this module will end and you will study new content which you will probably enjoy more.

It is essential that you understand your lectures, in order to achieve academic success. Therefore, if you are struggling to understand the content, first approach the lecturer and share how you feel. Remember, the lecturer can only help once they know there is a problem. The lecturer may provide extra notes or can spend some time explaining the content in more detail. Of course, it is always a good idea to take as many notes as you can, maybe recording the lecture, and perhaps comparing your notes with a friend. Asking each other questions to help clarify your understanding is a great way to help you process the information.

It may feel scary to show your vulnerability by asking your lecturer questions, however, remember you are at university to learn. Being able to say '*I don't understand*' is a sign of maturity as to how can you possibly know everything? A responsible student is one who appreciates they are not going to know everything immediately but with tenacity, practice, commitment and courage, you can persevere and take action to get the help and support you need and deserve. When you have reached success, you will feel so proud of yourself that you overcame the struggles you had.

It is easy to think it is all your responsibility that you are not understanding the content of the lecture, especially if you have your lecturer on a pedestal, such as if they are a professor, for example. However, it is also their responsibility to ensure they are pitching the content at the right level for you to understand. It may be that they may need to change how they deliver the content in order to suit your level of understanding. A good lecturer will check that their students understand what they are communicating; however, if this doesn't happen, then you have a right to say I don't understand. If you don't understand, it is likely there are other students who feel the same.

SELF-ENQUIRY REFLECTION 5.3

....

You are not expected to understand all the content from your lectures and seminars. However, there are strategies to help you and these questions will help you identify why you are struggling and what action you can take to help you understand the content better.

I have the courage to admit I am struggling to understand.

1. What content am I struggling to understand?

2. What are the reasons I am struggling to understand this lecture?

3. Which lectures do I understand?

4. What do I think the difference is between the lectures I understand and the ones I don't understand?

5. What action can I take to help me understand the lectures better?

LIFE LESSON

....

There will be times in your life when you struggle to understand the content of something and this is a normal part of any learning process. Admitting you don't understand something is courage in action as it is only then that you can take steps to find the answers.

TOPIC 5.4 I DON'T LIKE SPEAKING UP, EITHER ONLINE OR IN THE LECTURE HALL

Speaking up in lectures, either online or in person, can feel scary. This is because when you speak out in front of people, you are exposing yourself and therefore putting yourself in a position of vulnerability. You may have a fear of being laughed at and criticised by other students or a fear of being told you are wrong by your lecturer. To avoid looking stupid, it is easy to keep quiet and not speak up.

However, the empowering thing about feeling scared is that you can learn to overcome your fear. Once you realise you can handle speaking up and any consequences which may occur, the more resilient you will be. You learn you can handle being laughed at, criticised or told you are wrong (although it is very unlikely these things will happen).

The way you overcome your fears of speaking up is quite simple, you come out of your comfort zone and take a risk – you put yourself in a position to experience the situation you think you cannot handle. This is powerful because it is only when you realise you are not scared of something that it loses its power. Therefore, once you have spoken up and realised you can handle the consequences you are no longer scared of doing it. Of course, the first time you do it, you will feel ever so scared but what you will realise is, the world didn't end, simply because of how other people decided to react.

Technique 1: Affirmations of positivity

A great technique to use when doing something that scares you is to repeat a mantra in your head such as '*I can handle it*' or '*I've got this*' or '*All is good*' or '*I am safe*'. These affirmations of positivity validate you are not scared and therefore prevent that rush of adrenaline and cortisol – the hormones which are released when you are scared.

Technique 2: Leap of faith

Another great technique is to say to yourself, '*if not now then when*' as it is empowering to face your fears. Imagine leaving the lecture having spoken up compared to leaving the lecture after staying silent and inwardly berating yourself that you failed to speak up. Remember, confidence is built and enhanced with practice and university is a great place to learn social skills such as exerting your voice.

SELF-ENQUIRY REFLECTION 5.4

....

Speaking up in front of others can be extremely daunting, however like anything, the more you practice a task, the easier it becomes. These questions will help you become aware of your fears, helping you identify what you are really scared of.

I have the courage to speak up in front of others.

1. On a scale of 0–10 (10 being the maximum), how fearful am I of speaking up either in person or online in lectures or tutorials?

2. What do I think will happen if I speak up?

3. What are my specific fears in speaking up either in person or online?

4. What can I do to overcome my fears?

5. What resources, including people, could I use to help me feel confident speaking up more?

LIFE LESSON

....

Speaking up in front of people can seem challenging due to the feelings it can evoke within. However, being socially confident is an essential life skill and improves with practice. When you push through the uncomfortable pain of speaking up, you will realise your opinions matter and you are a great asset to the world.

TOPIC 5.5 I AM UNSURE HOW TO CHALLENGE THE VALIDITY OF WHAT I AM LEARNING

A fundamental aspect of learning in higher education is developing your ability to think for yourself. Throughout your university experience, you are encouraged to think critically including conducting your own research on a topic, usually in addition to what is being taught in lectures. This means thinking clearly and rationally about a subject and using your abilities to reason, analyse, debate and evaluate.

Critical thinking can mean you sometimes have to challenge the narrative you are being taught, which takes great courage and inner strength. It is important you do not allow your fear of upsetting others stop you from speaking your truth. Many people believe what they are told, simply because of the perceived position of authority of the person or platform sharing the information. However, it is important you question all ideas and assumptions rather than believing them at face value. The aim of critical thinking is to try to identify if the ideas, arguments and findings give you the whole picture or if there are inconsistencies in what you are being told.

Universities value students who can think critically as not only does it enhance your academic performance, but it is also an essential life skill to have after you leave university. This is because critical thinkers can demonstrate reasoning, evaluating, problem-solving, decision-making and analysis, which are all skills needed in your personal and professional life.

So how do you challenge the content which is being taught in your lectures or seminars? When you challenge, always start from a place of humility as there may be a chance you are not 100 per cent right. Therefore, have a mindset of curiosity and confidence – which means knowing you have a right to challenge, but keep an open mind. Having a positive intent behind your challenge to expand your knowledge means you, your lecturer and the student community will be able to explore alternative ideas.

You need to come out of your comfort zone when you challenge others, particularly those in authority yet, as with anything that feels scary, you need to be able to face your fear of getting 'told off' for questioning. Once you are familiar with challenging content, you become confident in doing it more often. Remember you are not challenging the lecturer but the content and have a right to do so.

SELF-ENQUIRY REFLECTION 5.5

. . . .

The more you challenge others in a positive way, the more you will be comfortable doing so. These questions will help you identify how you can improve your critical thinking skills, allowing you to challenge confidently and with curiosity.

I have the courage to positively challenge others.

1. On a scale of 0–10 (10 being the maximum), how confident am I challenging the content of what I am learning?

2. What may be stopping me from doing this?

3. What fears do I need to overcome to challenge more?

4. How can I become a better critical thinker in all areas of my life?

5. Who or what can you turn to for more support in becoming a better critical thinker?

LIFE LESSON

. . . .

Critical thinking and challenging other people's narratives are great skills to have, not only in your professional life but also in your personal life. Being able to make your own mind up after discerning the facts can protect you mentally, emotionally and financially. It is always a good idea to question what you are told by researching it for yourself. This includes being told something by a friend, family member, expert, the media, professional, government or any social platform.

TOPIC 5.6 HOW CAN I CREATE A SAFE, MOTIVATED PERSONAL SPACE FOR STUDYING?

Whether you are attending online lectures or need a private space to conduct your coursework, creating a conducive learning space is essential. Distractions can prevent you from committing to learning and these distractions can be in the form of people who want your time and energy, mobile phones pinging with messaging notifications and social media temptations. All these can prevent you from staying focused on the task at hand. Studying takes dedication and commitment and can sometimes be the hardest thing to do.

There are lots of great resources online which suggest ways of creating a great learning space – your university probably has its own guide. However, one of the best resources you can have are *boundaries*. This is when you have a set of guidelines or rules that you create, either for yourself or someone else. You create boundaries for several reasons such as helping you to achieve your goals, protect you emotionally and help you form healthy new habits.

Examples of great boundaries are:

- turning your phone off during study time;
- telling your friends to not contact you ensuring you are not going to be interrupted;
- setting a time limit for study then giving yourself a treat afterwards.

The university experience is one of taking responsibility and if you struggle to commit to your studies, then it is only you who is missing out and you deserve success. The more study you commit to, the better your chances are of finding work that you not only love but is financially rewarding. You have a right to shine in your career.

If you are unable to create an uninterrupted space in your living quarters then an alternative option may be to find another place to study which is quieter and with fewer interruptions. Also, think about what time is best for you to study – are you a morning or evening person?

However, it is also important you have balance in your life and some days you will feel less motivated to study and this is also okay. Have compassion for yourself and allow yourself some downtime to relax and have fun, which of course is all part of the university experience.

SELF-ENQUIRY REFLECTION 5.6

....

A safe uninterrupted study space is essential for academic success. These questions will help you identify how you can minimise interruptions meaning you commit to your study time enabling academic and personal success.

I have the courage to set boundaries with myself and others.

1. On a scale of 0–10 (10 being the maximum), how suitable is my study space?

2. What are my current interruptions and distractions?

3. How can I minimise these interruptions and distractions?

4. What boundaries do I need to have to help me commit to my study?

5. On the days I do not feel motivated to learn, what can I do to relax and chill?

LIFE LESSON

....

Learning to respect your need for your own space throughout your life is important for your well-being. Often, you can feel your energy being drained because of the people around you. If you learn to implement boundaries now, helping you to create a positive space, you will always be able to create an environment which supports your mental health.

TOPIC 5.7 HOW CAN I CREATE EFFECTIVE
PERSONAL TUTOR SESSIONS?

Every university student is assigned a personal tutor (sometimes called an academic adviser) and you will be expected to meet with them at least once during a semester, if not more. Their role is to focus on your academic and career goals and to help you navigate the higher education experience. They give feedback on your performance and help you identify your strengths and development areas to ensure study success. Working together with your tutor can mean you are more likely to achieve your full academic and personal potential and they are a great insider to have on your team.

Being able to have some time with an expert who can share their knowledge on assessment procedures, university regulations and module choices is a real gift. They can also help you think about life post graduation and can help identify future opportunities.

The sessions are a time for you to reflect and be honest about how you are feeling about your university experience and what you discuss is confidential between you both. If you can be as open as possible to receiving feedback, then this is a fantastic opportunity to identify not only how you can improve your academic abilities but also your overall mindset. Some may see this feedback as criticism, however, be reassured the intention of your tutor is to help you achieve your maximum potential and you can only improve if you know what needs improving.

You can also speak to your tutor about any personal challenges you are facing. You may think these are unrelated to your academic journey, but emotional challenges can stop you from focusing on your academic studies and therefore it is important to have support in this area. Your tutor is experienced in knowing the personal challenges which arise from studying and being away from home and will be able to share their wisdom to help you find peace with whatever is troubling you. Occasionally, they may need to refer you for more specialised support, and you should not see this as them rejecting you but simply wanting you to receive the best support and advice there is available.

It takes courage to trust a stranger and you may at first feel uncomfortable sharing how you feel; however, trust is built the more you learn the other person has your back. Once you can see your tutor has your best interests at heart you will be able to disclose how you feel and work together to attain the success you deserve.

SELF-ENQUIRY REFLECTION 5.7

Personal tutor sessions can help you achieve academic and personal success. These questions will help you identify your fears and benefits of attending personal tutor sessions, helping you to make a more informed choice. Accepting help is courage in action.

I have the courage to be honest and open with my tutor.

1. On a scale of 0–10 (10 being the maximum), how willing am I to attend my personal tutor sessions?

2. If this is below a 7, why am I considering not attending my personal tutor sessions?

3. What are my fears of attending the personal tutor sessions?

4. How would attending the sessions help me?
   (*Research the guidelines your university has regarding the personal tutor sessions they offer*)

5. On a scale of 0–10 (10 being the maximum), how willing are you to try at least *one* session to see how useful they will be for you?

LIFE LESSON

Many people are scared to ask for help as they think it is weak; however, the opposite is true. Asking for and being open to receiving wisdom from a more experienced person can help you to become the best version of yourself. In time, you will be able to share your knowledge to benefit others.

TOPIC 5.8 HOW DO I MAXIMISE
ONLINE LEARNING SUCCESS?

....

Many universities now offer online learning sessions which have been a huge transition for both tutors and students. Learning online is a different experience from learning in lecture halls and it can take time to adapt to this new way of learning. Some students prefer online learning and some really don't like it, however, being able to maximise the effectiveness of online learning is instrumental to your academic success.

Online learning is a lesson in courage as it can be scary for many reasons. Seeing yourself on screen throughout the lecture can be overwhelming. Therefore, some students choose to have the camera off while they are online. However, overcoming your fears is the only way to reduce feelings of discomfort and there will come a time in your work career when you must present with your camera on, so if you can overcome this fear now, then it bodes well for professional success.

Another great way to overcome your fear of online learning is to participate. It is very easy to hide behind the technology and not share your thoughts, especially if asked a question. Don't let your fear of speaking out stop you from engaging in the session. Participation helps you process your learning – and remember you are not expected to get everything right 100 per cent of the time and you are at university to learn. Using the chat functions and reaction tools are a great way to show that you want to participate, and your confidence will increase with practice.

Break-out rooms may be used in your online lecture, and this can also feel scary. Sharing your thoughts and opinions with people who you may not have met before can feel overwhelming. A great way to overcome this fear is to volunteer to speak first. I guarantee most people in the break-out group will be as nervous as you and will welcome your courage. The feeling you will have after you have used your courage to speak out is addictive, as you realise you are a confident soul after all.

Learning online is a new skill to conquer and the more you can push through your fears, the more comfortable you will feel as it becomes the norm. Your university will have an online learning guide to help you maximise online learning success meaning you obtain the grades you deserve.

SELF-ENQUIRY REFLECTION 5.8

....

Online learning is a very different experience from classroom teaching. Adapting to this method can take time. These questions will help you reflect on what you dislike and how you can increase your confidence meaning you achieve the success you deserve.

I have the courage to participate in online learning.

1. On a scale of 0–10 (10 being the maximum), how confident am I attending online learning?

2. What do I dislike about online learning?

3. What fears are stopping me from getting the best from online learning?

4. What do I like about online learning?

5. How can I become comfortable with online learning?

LIFE LESSON

....

Being confident to speak up online is a skill you will need for your professional life. Learning to be confident now using this intervention will help you achieve the academic and professional success you deserve. The more you '*Feel the fear and do it anyway®*' (Jeffers, 1987) the more confident you will be in using digital communication interventions.

CHAPTER 6
COMPLETING COURSE WORK AND ASSIGNMENTS

....

Challenges are what makes life interesting and overcoming them is what makes life meaningful.

Author unknown

SCENARIO

....

Tanya woke with a start and wondered what the constant banging noise was. Realising Ellie, her partner, was not beside her in bed, she figured she must be already up and entertaining Seb, their eight-month-old. Feeling both grateful and guilty that she had managed to get a lie-in, Tanya jumped out of bed and rushed downstairs to relieve Ellie of parenting duties.

Ellie smiled as Tanya walked through the door, pleased she had managed a sleep in and feeling blessed they had met over 10 years ago. Their relationship had solid foundations and they never exchanged angry words with each other, managing to work through any challenges with honest communication and the intent of wanting each other to be happy.

'*Sorry El, I didn't mean to sleep in so late*', sighed Tanya, grabbing a cup and filling it up with coffee from the espresso machine.

'*Hey, you needed it after all that late night study*', replied Ellie as she wiped baby food off Sebastian's chin.

Ellie was aware Tanya had crawled into bed past midnight after she had spent all day writing an assignment which had to be submitted in three days.

After spending all day at the library, Tanya had tried to summarise her research early evening after she had finished Seb's night-time routine but was so exhausted she had spent a large proportion of her time, staring at the screen not knowing what to write, resulting in her getting distracted on Instagram and TikTok. She had finally retired to bed exhausted, yet unable to sleep.

Once again, Tanya wondered why she was putting herself through this Master's degree, worrying about the debt she was accruing and the pressure she was putting on their relationship as Tanya had to pay the bills and look after Seb.

'*Stop it!*' said Ellie firmly, looking across at Tanya. '*I know what you are doing – guilt tripping yourself about this course and we have talked about it, it's fine, we will manage, and it will be worth it when you have passed.*'

Tanya smiled gratefully at Ellie, amazed at how she seemed to know what was going through her mind.

'*Do you really think I can do it?*' asked Tanya, seeking the reassurance she needed to hear. '*I mean, this assignment has to be handed in on Wednesday and I am struggling to finish it. I have a presentation to do the following Friday which is making me feel sick and I nearly failed my last module. You know El, maybe it is time to call it a day. I mean, who do I think I am?*' added Tanya mournfully.

Ellie gently fastened Seb into his bouncer, turned on the timer and after ensuring he was settled, grabbed herself a coffee, and led Tanya over to the settee.

'*Tan, look at me,*' asserted Ellie.

> *I need you to stop this self-sabotage. This is not your voice, it's just a story you are telling yourself, rooted in crappy fear and self-doubt. Stop expecting yourself to be perfect. You are doing amazingly well: you gave birth to Seb only eight months ago, have adapted brilliantly to motherhood, you work part-time, are supporting your sister with cancer, managing your dad's dementia, and are completing a Master's degree for god's sake. Please give yourself some credit for how strong you are being.*

Ellie burst into tears, even though she was immensely grateful for Tanya's support she just felt so overwhelmed and anxious with everything these days and didn't know what to do.

Remember ... you've got this

Academic study can be a test of your tenacity, mental willpower and emotional strength. Faced with learning new subjects and developing the skills to research, debate and critically argue can challenge any student, no matter how intelligent you are. In addition, having to manage your studies around the rest of your life can make you feel overwhelmed and anxious at times.

However, overcoming challenges such as these can empower you to believe in yourself as you realise you are stronger than you think you are. Adversity helps you to develop trust and faith in yourself that you can handle more than you ever thought you could. This builds emotional resilience and confidence as you realise you can deal with current challenges and any future ones which may arise. You realise you were good enough all along.

Academic study can be particularly challenging at times, for example receiving lower marks than you expected, working in groups with people who irritate you, dealing with friends who receive better marks than you or having to deliver presentations; all of which can trigger feelings of insecurity. However, learning to face all these situations is part of academic life and you will soon realise you can and will handle it all.

If you accept your academic journey is going to have highs and lows yet commit to learning from everything that happens to you, you can make every experience empowering, building a healthy love and respect for yourself.

When you start to ask, 'What is this experience teaching me?' instead of 'Why is this happening to me?' life becomes a rich adventure.

Learning from experiences means you look for life lessons.

- If you fail a module, ask how can I do better next time?
- If you fear asking for help, dig deep to discover why this is.
- If you hate presenting, question what precisely are you scared of.

COMPLETING COURSE WORK AND ASSIGNMENTS

- If you easily get distracted, challenge yourself to commit.
- If you want to give up, remember why you started.

Nobody is perfect and everyone struggles in life sometimes yet facing adversity at university teaches you how to be strong, kind and gentle with yourself and realise you can resiliently handle all the university experience has to offer.

Remember, you are worthy and deserving of receiving your degree.

TOPIC 6.1 | I DON'T KNOW WHERE TO START IN COMPLETING MY ASSIGNMENT

Starting assignments can appear a monumental task, especially if you are struggling to understand the question. Your uncertainty and confusion can make you feel overwhelmed and anxious meaning you procrastinate. This means you busy yourself with anything else rather than focusing on the assignment and as the submission date looms closer, you may panic.

Procrastination is rooted in fear, and it is therefore helpful to identify what you are fearing. Is it a fear of getting it wrong, a fear of failure, a fear of low grades or simply a more practical fear of wondering how you are going to complete 3000 words on a subject you are struggling to understand?

Once you have identified your fear, consider if you are striving for perfection, which is also rooted in fear. Perfectionism can stop you from starting your work, but perfection doesn't exist so don't let this illusion hold you back. Remind yourself that good enough is good enough. Whatever your fears are, the important thing is to address them and not allow them to have control over you.

The best way to face any fears is by taking action. Begin by naming the challenge you are facing regarding starting your work, list the solution and finally determine the action.

EXAMPLE

Challenge: I don't know where to start in writing my assignment.
Solution: Ask someone who can help me start the assignment.
Action: Email my lecturer on Monday to ask for help.

You may be fearful of reaching out for help due to feeling embarrassed but remember you are learning to become a researcher and academic writer, and this takes time and practice. Receiving help is an essential part of your development so be kind to yourself. Receiving feedback on your writing style helps you improve. If your initial submissions were not well received, trust you will become more proficient as you gain experience.

Your university or department is likely to have an online guide to help you write assignments and many offer study skills courses through the learning resource centre. Although attending these events can take time, they can provide helpful advice and tips to help you start your assignments. And remember if you don't start, you will never have the joy and satisfaction of completing and handing in your work.

COMPLETING COURSE WORK AND ASSIGNMENTS

SELF-ENQUIRY REFLECTION 6.1

....

Identifying the reason for your procrastination is key to starting your work. These questions will help you identify what is stopping you and how you can overcome these fears, meaning you can take action to complete the task at hand.

I have the courage to start my assignment.

1. What is stopping me from starting my assignment including specific fears I have?

2. List the *solutions* and the *actions* I can take to overcome the answers I have written to question 1.

3. Give an example of a time in the past when I overcame something I struggled to start.

4. How did I overcome this in the past and how can I apply the same strategies now?

5. What resources can I use to help me complete my assignment?
   (*lecturer, student support, tutor, online guides, friends, forums*)

LIFE LESSON

....

There may be times in your life when you procrastinate about starting something. However, at the root of procrastination is fear and therefore identifying your fears can help you move forward. The more you take action to overcome your fears, the more confident you will feel as you realise how internally strong you really are.

TOPIC 6.2 I AM FRIGHTENED OF FAILING AT UNIVERSITY

Worries about failing may be negatively affecting your university experience. You may stress about not achieving good grades and this may trigger insecurities within. However, attending university is more than just obtaining good grades – it is also about having fun, creating memories, sharing good times, increasing your resilience, becoming self-aware and learning to become independent.

You may put yourself under immense pressure to obtain top grades and when you don't, you may berate and criticise yourself, meaning you suffer mentally. Instead, try congratulating yourself for trying so hard and courageously traversing this new academic experience. You tried your best and this needs to be acknowledged. Sometimes other responsibilities can stop you from dedicating as much time as you wanted, but this is okay too. If you know deep down, you didn't commit as much as you could have, then learn from this and commit more next time.

Not only can a fear of failing make you worry, but it can also stop you from embracing all that life has to offer. You may stay in your comfort zone, which means you don't take positive risks, meaning you miss out on new opportunities. However, if you learn to face your fears, you will be open to things which can enhance your life.

EXAMPLE

How fears can limit opportunity

Imagine you have been asked to present your research at a conference but your fears of getting it wrong and blushing stop you from accepting this opportunity. You stay in your comfort zone and decline this invitation, watching a fellow student present instead. Later you learn she was approached by a representative from a large multi-national organisation who had attended the conference and was offered an internship. This could have been you, but your fears stopped you from benefiting from this amazing opportunity.

Examine the risks you have overcome so far in your life.

- You learnt to walk and talk.
- You attended school and college.
- You passed exams.

- You made friends.
- You tried new hobbies.
- You applied to and attended university.

These are all calculated risks you took and overcame, although you may have failed along the way while taking these risks, the failures helped empower you to be the person you are today. If you believe it is okay to fail and face your fears, then you can learn to embrace and overcome them, leading to success.

SELF-ENQUIRY REFLECTION 6.2

....

Welcoming failure means you are a confident person, not scared of failing so it holds no power over you. You become empowered by trying new experiences which push you out of your comfort zone. You become resilient as you do not see failure as a shameful event but as an experience which helps you grow.

I have the courage to face my fear of failure.

1. On a scale of 0–10 (10 being the maximum), how scared am I of failure?

2. Where do I think I learned to fear failing?

3. If I reframe failure as a positive event, how does failure empower me?

4. What am I saying no to because of my fear of failure?

5. What action can I take to start to overcome my fear of failure?

LIFE LESSON

....

Using courage to overcome your fears means you embrace new opportunities which increase your confidence, resulting in great mental health. If you find yourself wanting to do something but making excuses, take the time to name your fears and take action to overcome them. You deserve happiness and success.

TOPIC 6.3 I FEEL ANXIOUS ABOUT SUBMITTING MY WORK

You have spent hours completing your assignment and now it is finally submission day. After your intense effort, you may welcome this day or may feel a deep sense of dread.

The resistance you feel may be your mind telling you a story that your work is not good enough and you need to spend more time on it. However, this negative narrative can be rooted in perfectionism, which is fearful thinking, perhaps because you are worried you will not achieve high marks. Your negative thoughts trigger a biological response meaning adrenaline and cortisol flood your body, resulting in physical feelings often called anxiety.

The way to overcome this is to reframe your thoughts into positive thoughts and become your own best friend – support yourself like you would your best friend.

EXAMPLE

Your friend has spent a great deal of time and effort on their work. However, they have called you to tell you they don't want to submit it as they think it is not good enough. What supportive and inspirational words would you offer them?

Now imagine saying these supportive words to yourself.

This is a powerful psychological process as when you focus on another person, you disassociate from your emotions and fears, allowing you to use your logical, strategic thinking part of your brain. Hopefully, you have spoken some positive words to yourself and feel a little calmer now.

It is also important you appreciate how hard you have worked and the commitment you have shown to your studies, submitting your work is recognition of this process. The university experience can be demanding so show yourself compassion. How can you be kind and gentle with yourself regarding all your hard work?

Anxiety is another word for fear, therefore if you still are afraid about submitting your work, identify what your fears are. It may be familiar fears of failing, getting it wrong or being criticised. However, the only way to overcome these fears is to face them. Submitting your work is the best way to face your fears as you realise, your fears have no power over you anymore.

Receiving feedback is recognition of your hard work and helps you progress in your studies to get the results you deserve. Remember you are at university to learn, so it is okay to take the pressure off yourself and learn from the constructive feedback which will be given. You are not expected to be perfect – there is no such thing.

SELF-ENQUIRY REFLECTION 6.3

. . . .

Being vulnerable enough to receive feedback aids your personal and professional development. Yes, you may be fearful of receiving poor feedback; however, no feedback is poor if it teaches you how to improve at something. These questions will help you see the benefits of submitting your work.

I have the courage to submit my work.

1. On a scale of 0–10, how fearful am I of submitting my work?

2. If I had to name my fears regarding submission, what do I think I am fearful about?

3. What are the benefits of submitting my work?

4. What kind words can I say to myself to help me overcome the negative chatter in my head about submitting my work?

5. What can I learn from the feedback I receive?

LIFE LESSON

. . . .

Receiving critical feedback can be upsetting, especially if you are questioning your knowledge and ability. However, feedback is a gift if it's from a source that is supportive and wants to help you. Have the courage to ask for feedback but discern if the feedback is from someone who is in a trustworthy position to give it to you.

TOPIC 6.4 I AM STRUGGLING TO WRITE MY ASSIGNMENT AND NO ONE ELSE IS

If you are struggling to write your assignment, it is easy to think no one else feels the same way. However, many students feel stuck and confused like you, but don't want to admit it due to a fear of being inadequate. The more you believe your fear-based story, that it is only you who is struggling, the more negative thoughts you will experience, ultimately creating feelings of anxiety and panic.

Continual negative thoughts trigger chemical hormones into your bloodstream which make you feel even more anxious. However, there is an easy way to stop this: seek out evidence which contradicts the story you are telling yourself.

A simple psychological process can help you switch the negative story which is creating unease to one which is much more supportive, inspiring and factual.

EXAMPLE

Eliminate the negative chatter in your head

1. Write down the story you are telling yourself about the current situation. (For example, I am the only person struggling to complete this assignment.)
2. Ask yourself, what evidence do you have that what you have written is true? If you were in front of a judge in a courtroom, could you prove your story with facts, logic and reason? (For example, how do you know no one else is struggling?)
3. Seek out and present any evidence to discredit your negative story. (For example, your closest friend said they are confused too.)

In the example above, you might think others appear to understand the assignment, yet you may have no evidence at all to support this hypothesis. Perhaps by asking other students you will learn they too are struggling. You may also ask your lecturer or tutor if past students have struggled and receive confirmation they have. These are examples of seeking evidence to discredit your fear-based story.

Once you understand the stories in your head dictate your reality, you realise how powerful you are because you can create a new story filled with positive thoughts and actions you can take to succeed.

Take control of the story in your head and you will feel much better, both mentally and emotionally.

SELF-REFLECTION EXERCISE 6.4

. . . .

Becoming aware of your worries helps you realise how much fear is impacting your life. Fear can stand for *False Evidence Appearing Real* and realising your story is fake can stop your anxious feelings. These questions will help you understand how much your fake fear-based stories are negatively impacting your life.

I have the courage to let go of fake stories I am telling myself.

1. On a scale of 0–10 (10 being the maximum), how good am I at telling myself fake stories which I don't have any evidence for?

2. Detail an example of a negative story I once told myself and how later I found out it was untrue.

3. When I told myself this negative story, how did it make me feel?

4. What story am I telling myself now and how much factual evidence do I have that it is true?

5. What evidence do I need to discredit the story I am telling myself to help me feel better?

LIFE LESSON

. . . .

Throughout life, you may tell yourself fake stories about situations which, on reflection, you realise have no supporting evidence. Learn to challenge these unhelpful narratives and you will feel calmer, more in control and able to make more empowered decisions. Ask questions to help gain evidence helping you to disprove any negative narrative you are telling yourself.

TOPIC 6.5 I DON'T WANT TO ASK MY LECTURER FOR HELP AS I MAY GET MARKED DOWN

This is a common belief and explains why some students struggle in silence, scared to ask their lecturer for help. However, it is important to understand that academic staff are on your side and are committed to your success. You may believe it is a lack of intelligence which makes you struggle to understand the content; however, you may have a different way of learning facts from others, including your lecturer, and this is okay. We all process information differently and can benefit from one-to-one teaching to help understand the content.

It may also be that you generally don't like asking people for help as you believe it is weak.

Reflect on the following.

1. How willing am I to ask people for help?
2. Do I see asking for help as a strength or a weakness?
3. Do I think I should be able to do everything on my own?
4. Are people who ask for help confident or weak?
5. What are the benefits of asking for help?
6. How do I feel when someone asks me for help?

Being able to ask others for help is a strength, not a weakness. Of course, it is important that you exercise independence and aim to be responsible for yourself in life as much as you can. However, sometimes is it important to reach out for help to someone who has more wisdom and experience on a subject.

Your lecturer wants to see you evolve and grow which includes you being able to ask for help. This then allows you to become more competent in a subject. You are not going to be marked down simply for seeking clarification on a subject if it will help you understand it at a deeper level. If you demonstrate that you have committed to your studies and have started to research the subject but are still struggling, then the lecturer will be more than willing to help you.

The first step in reaching out for help is to be clear about what help you need and the specific answers you are seeking. Write a list of the clarity you need, to be able to complete your work. If you are struggling to know what to research, then ask for guidance on this as a starting point. Once you are clear on this then contact the person who can help you.

Remember you are at university to learn and part of learning is not knowing. You only become competent by admitting what you don't know. It takes courage to admit you don't know something and not knowing does not mean you are a failure; it means you are ready, willing and able to learn.

SELF-REFLECTION EXERCISE 6.5

....

Admitting you don't know something is courageous and the more you can do this, the more you are open to learning. These questions will help you identify what is stopping you from asking for help. Self-care is reaching out to others for support.

I have the courage to admit I don't know the answer.

1. On a scale of 0–10, how comfortable am I in asking for help in different areas of my life?

2. What stops me from asking for help from others?

3. What would be the benefits of asking for help?

4. What is stopping me from asking for help from the lecturer?

5. What would be the benefits of asking for help from the lecturer?

LIFE LESSON

....

The more comfortable you become in asking others for help, the more you are willing to receive it. If you try to deal with everything alone, this can negatively impact your mental health. It takes courage to admit you need help and reach out to others for it.

TOPIC 6.6 I WANT TO GIVE UP WHEN I DON'T RECEIVE THE MARKS I HAD HOPED FOR

You may feel pressured to achieve the highest grades possible while studying at university. This pressure can feel burdensome, often resulting in increased panic and anxiety. Yet it can be unrealistic to expect to receive high marks consistently, especially with first submissions or subjects you are unfamiliar with or don't like.

It may also be that others in your life expect you to receive high marks and if you don't, their criticism and judgement can make you feel unworthy and not good enough. However, they are not you and not experiencing university life so show yourself compassion and kindness for your efforts, not only now but throughout the rest of your life.

It is common to put pressure on yourself to achieve in all areas of your life – to be perfect in all ways. (However, there is no such thing as perfection.) Your school experience sets an expectation to get high marks, and anything less is seen as failure. Unfortunately, this can create a behavioural pattern of having perfectionist expectations and over-trying which can create internal stress. The way to overcome this is to reassure yourself that it is okay to get the right grades for you at this moment in time. Allowing yourself to simply *pass* a module if you are finding it hard is okay and a good way to avoid burnout.

Remember your studies are just one area of your university experience, and you will excel in other ways. You are at university to learn lots of things, not just your ability to memorise facts or argue a piece of research. The practical and social skills you learn are just as important and seeing the opportunities in experiences may guide you in a different direction than what you expected.

For example, you may receive low marks in your law degree module on land law, yet cooking for yourself you realise you love it and decide you want to open your own restaurant one day. Perhaps cooking is your passion and law was simply a subject which you liked at school.

Give yourself permission to commit to your studies 100 per cent yet still enjoy the whole of the university experience. If you leave university a more evolved, conscious, aware individual, knowing where your passion lies, this can be better than leaving with the highest marks in a subject which barely holds your interest anymore.

SELF-REFLECTION EXERCISE 6.6

. . . .

It is understandable you would like to obtain high marks; however, ask yourself why? This desire may be rooted in a story you are telling yourself that you will only be good enough if you achieve the highest marks possible, yet on deeper reflection, this is an illusion as you are good enough regardless.

I have the courage to be proud of whatever grades I achieve.

1. On a scale of 0–10, 10 being the maximum, how much am I pushing myself to achieve the highest marks possible?

2. What are my reasons for wanting to get the highest marks possible?

3. How may this pressure be affecting me?

4. If I don't receive the highest marks possible, what will I tell myself?

5. How can I still reassure myself that I am good enough even if I don't receive the highest marks possible?

LIFE LESSON

. . . .

Learning to know when you are pushing yourself excessively is important for good mental health. Knowing when and how to balance all areas of your life is key to living an enjoyable life. Allowing yourself to be gentle with yourself is essential for personal and professional success.

TOPIC 6.7 I GET EASILY DISTRACTED WHEN RESEARCHING AND WRITING ASSIGNMENTS

Finding the motivation to complete assignments can be an ongoing struggle at university. Appreciate there are going to be occasions when you would rather do anything else. Practice self-compassion as you can't expect to be motivated 100 per cent of the time.

When you are demotivated, it is easy to get distracted. Sometimes you are de-motivated because you do now know what to write and if this is the case, then seeking help is important. Who can you ask for help?

However, you may also be unfocused due to:

- a new relationship;
- ongoing emotional dramas in your life;
- opportunities to experience more fun things than academic study;
- feeling tired and overwhelmed;
- different demands being placed on you and suffering from burnout;
- lack of interest in the subject.

Whatever your distraction, it is important you identify why you are de-motivated and what obstacles are stopping you from completing the work. This means taking personal responsibility and part of this process is calling yourself out when you are not acting in a responsible and empowered way. Admit when you are not committing 100 per cent and resolve to remove the obstacles which are stopping you from committing to your studies.

Having strong boundaries can help manage distractions, for example:

- turn off notifications and put your phone out of reach;
- ask people not to interrupt you;
- find a place where you can study without being interrupted;
- ensure you are not hungry or thirsty before you start;
- create a plan of what you intend to complete in your study time.

Implementing the above boundaries will help you complete and submit your work.

However, it is also important you listen to how you feel mentally, emotionally and physically. It may be that you are exhausted for various reasons, and you simply do not have the energy to complete your work. If you feel this way, it is important to rest and even consider applying for a submission extension.

SELF-ENQUIRY REFLECTION 6.7

....

Being able to commit to your studies in the time you have allocated helps you then enjoy your free time. These questions will help you understand what your distractions are and how you can minimise them to help focus on your studies.

I have the courage to commit to my academic work.

1. On a scale of 0–10, how easily do I get distracted from studying?

2. What distracts me?

3. How can I take responsibility to minimise these distractions? (*think about any boundaries you can set with yourself and others*)

4. How would an empowered, motivated person behave when completing the assignment?

5. How have I been getting in my own way and not committing to my studies? (*Have compassion for yourself when writing this answer, it is not an excuse to mentally beat yourself with a stick*)

LIFE LESSON

....

Distractions and lack of motivation can apply in any area of your life but being able to identify why you are distracted and demotivated can help you form a plan of action to overcome these issues. Tenacity is a skill to develop and can help you achieve both personally and professionally. Be kind to yourself – no one is motivated 100 per cent of the time.

TOPIC 6.8 I HAVE RECEIVED LOW MARKS
AND DON'T KNOW WHY

Receiving low marks after you have worked hard can feel disappointing. You may feel like you want to give up, you may be angry with your lecturer and even wonder if there is any point in continuing. These are all understandable reactions when faced with this situation. However, remind yourself of the hard work you committed to and feel proud of your achievement, regardless of the mark.

Before you start to berate yourself, ask yourself, are my grades really that poor or are they simply not what I expected or wanted? It is human nature to want the best grade but sometimes this is not always realistic and having more manageable expectations is a sign of self-love and maturity.

Allow yourself to feel disappointed yet remember you may have been conditioned by previous experiences, such as school to achieve a top mark. However, university is not only about obtaining high marks but learning to be an academic writer and enjoying the process of becoming independent and maturing as an individual.

If you have received low marks and are confused about why, make it a priority to seek feedback from your lecturer. This is part of their role; to ensure you learn from your work, enabling you to achieve better marks next time. Although it can be painful, it is also enlightening as you realise how you can improve next time.

It may also be that on this occasion you simply did not connect with the subject matter and were disinterested. You cannot be passionate about every module on your course.

Not many people like to fail against the standards they set themselves, and your ego may have been bruised. However, acknowledging you feel disappointed and hurt, but being able to move on is a sign of maturity. In addition, reflecting on what you have learned from achieving low grades also helps you gain better marks moving forward.

It is also important to seek out solace and comfort from someone who is on your team, who can offer kindness and encouragement. Try to avoid those who may criticise you as this will make you feel worse.

Finally, remember to keep this situation in perspective, this is just one module or one assignment where you have not achieved the marks you want. It is a small blip in your life and one which you will barely remember in ten years.

SELF-ENQUIRY REFLECTION 6.8

....

Not achieving the marks you want can be disheartening and knock your confidence. However, the grades you receive do not mean you are inadequate, and it is important to keep this in perspective. If you committed 100 per cent and tried your best, then that is certainly good enough. Look at the bigger picture of your whole university experience.

I have the courage to bounce back after low marks.

1. How am I feeling after receiving low marks?

2. What do I need right now and from whom?

3. If I am confused about receiving low marks, how can I gain clarity?

4. How can I be kinder to myself regarding receiving these marks?

5. How would I cheer up a friend who had tried hard but obtained low marks?

LIFE LESSON

....

There may be times in your life when you will feel disappointed such as not achieving a job or promotion, and this is okay. Being able to allow yourself to feel disappointed is an act of self-compassion. There is always something to learn from events which do not turn out as you wanted them to. Trust there is a bigger picture to your life which has not been fully revealed yet.

TOPIC 6.9 I FEEL ENVIOUS OF FRIENDS WHO HAVE RECEIVED BETTER GRADES THAN ME

It is understandable to feel upset when your friends receive higher grades than you. To feel envy is a human emotion so do not berate yourself for feeling this way. Envy is simply a longing for something that you want. You can use envy in a positive way to re-focus on what you want to achieve in your life.

You can feel envious and still be a good friend – both can be true. Yet a productive way to use envy in this context is to use it to motivate you to understand yourself and the subject better next time. You may also be balancing other demands in your life and cannot commit the time needed to get the results you want. Being able to manage all areas of your life and still ensure your mental health is in good shape is much more important than achieving the highest grades possible.

It is also important to be aware of the differences between you and your friend. Maybe you are having relationship difficulties or work part time and your friend doesn't. Maybe your friend is a perfectionist, and you are not. This is good as it means you do not put as much pressure on yourself resulting in better mental health. It is important you do not think you are inferior to your friend in any way but accept you are two different people on two different journeys.

Comparing yourself to another in any area of your life is a waste of your valuable energy and can make you feel inadequate and insecure. You have unique gifts which in time you will see. Obtaining a low grade on a piece of work does not take anything away from you as an individual. Have confidence that you did the best you could do and the grades you have obtained at this point in time are unlikely to have a huge effect on your future success. Resilience comes from learning it is okay to fail or get low marks, at least you passed!

Accept what you can achieve right now and be proud of what you are achieving in every area of your life, not just this one. Allowing yourself to be proud of all that you have achieved is a sign of self-love.

So, congratulate your friend, reassure yourself how well you are doing and commit to your studies. This is just one situation from which you can learn. When you stop comparing yourself to another, you reclaim your personal power.

SELF-ENQUIRY REFLECTION 6.9

....

Comparing your achievements to another can be destructive to your self-esteem and mental health. Being able to detach from others and focus on yourself and your own life goals is important for your well-being as you have your own path to walk. These questions will help you understand your feelings.

I have the courage to feel disappointment and envy.

1. On a scale of 0–10 (10 being the maximum), how upset and envious do I feel when my friends receive better grades than me?

2. What is it that upsets me about this situation?

3. How can I allow myself to feel these emotions?

4. How can I be kinder to myself in this situation?

5. How can I use this experience to better myself in any way?

LIFE LESSON

....

Comparing yourself to your friends or other people can be a waste of time and energy. Always ask yourself, what can I learn from this, rather than using your resentment and envy as a stick to beat yourself with. Trust you have a path to follow which may be different from others.

TOPIC 6.10 I DISAGREE WITH MY GRADES EVEN AFTER RECEIVING FEEDBACK

....

You may have received lower marks than what you were expecting, and after obtaining feedback from the lecturer, still feel confused regarding how you could have improved and obtained a better mark. It may be a good idea to arrange a meeting with your tutor to discuss this matter further. They may be able to offer you an objective view and help you see the situation in a different way, gain clarity for you or even explain the process to appeal the grade.

If you are still unhappy after this meeting a more formal appeal may be needed and your university will have a complaints and appeals procedure which will be available on your university website. If you cannot find this, speak to student services for further advice and guidance as you will not be the first person to have experienced this.

You may be fearful of taking this more formal approach; however, standing up for yourself is part of being a mature, independent and empowered individual. Everyone has the right to do this including you.

Challenging perceived authority can be scary as you may have been told from a young age to 'do as you are told'. While this may have been the truth when you were a child, it is certainly not the reality now you are an adult. Being able to express your needs politely yet firmly can help increase your self-belief. This is a time for you to protect yourself and no one else can do it for you. You may win the appeal, or you may receive different feedback which will help you gain better marks next time.

If you feel uncomfortable while following the appeals and complaints procedure, ensure you have support from someone. Don't think you are causing trouble in some way: it is sensible to resolve this situation through the correct channels rather than forever feeling resentful about the grade you received and knowing you didn't challenge it because of your fear.

Of course, appealing a grade should only be used when you are genuinely confused as to why you obtained the grade you did. Standing up for yourself is a sign of being authentic and is a great quality to embody.

SELF-ENQUIRY REFLECTION 6.10

....

Being assertive and standing up for what you believe in is important, not only while you are at university but throughout the rest of your life. These questions will help you explore why you are resistant to doing this and help you overcome any blockages you have.

I have a right to appeal the grades I have received.

1. On a scale from 0–10 (10 being the maximum), how much do I believe I have received an unfair grade?

2. How has the feedback I received fail to reassure me that my mark was accurate?

3. On a scale of 0–10 (10 being the maximum), how comfortable am I in using the appeals and complaint procedure?

4. What are my fears in using this procedure?

5. How can I overcome my fears and who can help me do this?

LIFE LESSON

....

Challenging perceived authority is often needed in life. Remember, just because someone is in a position of power does not mean they have your best interests at heart or are right. Being able to stand up for yourself and your loved ones is a form of mental and emotional protection and is essential for good mental well-being.

TOPIC 6.11 I AM DUE TO DELIVER A PRESENTATION BUT FEEL ANXIOUS

The thought of delivering presentations can make you feel scared or anxious. This is because you experience fear when you are uncertain about an outcome. Presenting to others always has an unknown outcome, yet the more presentations you deliver the more confident you will become as you realise you can handle anything that happens when presenting.

There may be voice in your head which can be sabotaging you. It may be saying things like:

- I will get it wrong and forget what I am going to say;
- I may go red and feel embarrassed;
- I may not know the answers to questions.

These are all understandable thoughts which are fear based, creating the feelings of anxiety, and, yes, some of them may even come true. However, a key component of overcoming fear is knowing you can handle whatever happens and the more presentations you deliver, the more experienced you will become, and your anxiety will reduce.

The following points may help reduce your anxiety.

- Prepare well, know your subject and be passionate about it.
- Don't expect yourself to be perfect – there is no such thing.
- See presenting as a continual learning experience in which you will improve each time.

In addition, reflect on the benefits presenting will give you. You may learn you love giving presentations and want to make it your career, or realise it is a great experience for when you present in your job. Delivering presentations is a skill that needs practice so don't expect yourself to be a top-class presenter at first.

It is okay to be scared about giving presentations as you are at your most vulnerable; however, knowing you can handle being vulnerable and yet still survive helps you have faith in yourself and your abilities. Repeating '*I can handle it*' when you are about to start your presentation can help calm your anxious mind.

SELF-ENQUIRY REFLECTION 6.11

· ·

Being asked to present at university can provoke fear but learning to overcome your fear means your anxiety reduces. Be kind to yourself and know that it is okay to feel this way and know that overcoming fears is key to becoming more confident.

I have the courage to overcome my fears about presenting.

1. On a scale of 0–10 (10 being the maximum), how scared am I of delivering presentations?

2. What are my top three fears about presenting?

3. How much experience do I have in delivering presentations?

4. What would a wise kind supportive person say about how I am feeling about presenting?

5. What action can I take to ensure I deliver an awesome presentation? (*prepare well, practice, know my subject, practice presenting to friends/family*)

LIFE LESSON

· · · · · · · · · · · · · · · · · ·

Delivering presentations either in person or online is a key component of many job roles, therefore the more practice you have at university the better. Being passionate when you present reassures the audience you know your subject which builds your confidence. In time, as your experience grows, you will feel more reassured regarding your presentation skills.

TOPIC 6.12 I AM WORKING IN A GROUP AND STRUGGLING TO GET ON WITH MY PEERS

Group work is expected throughout the university experience and is good practice for working as part of a team in your future career. However, some people struggle with group work because of the different personality types and the dynamics at play. Accepting this and knowing it is okay to feel this way means you can learn to manage the situation better.

Working in groups can trigger you emotionally. For example, there may be a bossy person who tells you what to do or someone who doesn't seem to do their fair share of the work. Think about why you are giving your power away and getting triggered by another. You do not want another person to be able to have control of your emotions in this way so reflect on why you are getting triggered. You cannot expect another to change their behaviour, but you can modify your own, choose not to react and exhibit self-control. You may get emotionally triggered as you are doubting yourself and your abilities in some way. The other group members may seem to know the subject more or are spending more time on the project than you can. Be kind and gentle with yourself; are you performing to the best of your knowledge and ability? You may not have as much time as they have due to managing other demands in your life. Speak kindly to yourself about how well you are doing.

Maybe this group situation will teach you the art of accepting others. You will not have to work with these people forever – it will pass – so accept you cannot get along with everyone. You may be the type of person who prefers working independently and this is okay too.

Knowing your boundaries is another good way to manage group work. For example, due to other commitments, you may not be able to spend as much time on the work as some members of the group. Being able to communicate these limitations is essential in the group process. If you are delegated a piece of work by another group member which you don't feel happy with, have the courage to say how you feel. Group work can be a great exercise in learning to be assertive.

If group work is really making you uncomfortable, speak to your tutor who may be able to offer some wise advice. Equally just airing your frustrations can help you feel better about the situation. This is only one module out of your whole university experience, and it will pass.

SELF-ENQUIRY REFLECTION 6.12

. . . .

Group work can be a struggle especially when other people fail to commit their time and energy which can affect your grade. However, it is a great opportunity to practice asserting your needs, practise patience and the art of compromise.

I have the courage to handle group work.

1. On a scale of 0–10 (10 being the maximum), how challenging am I finding group work?

2. What is causing my pain?

3. What is this group work experience teaching me about myself?
   (*I need to have more patience, tolerance, accept differences, assert myself, say no*)

4. How can I take responsibility to improve the group work experience?

5. How can I speak kindly to myself while I am experiencing this?

LIFE LESSON

. . . .

Not letting other people's personalities affect you is an ongoing life lesson. There will always be people you do not resonate with but may have to work with them in some capacity. People view the world differently based on their level of consciousness and knowing this means you can have compassion for yourself and others.

CHAPTER 7
PASSING EXAMS AND SUCCESSFUL REVISION

....

To conquer fear is the beginning of wisdom

Bertrand Russell

SCENARIO

....

Milo yawned and despondently looked at his revision notes scattered in front of him. Glancing at the clock, he was shocked to see it showed 3am; no wonder he felt so exhausted, but still something inside him would not let him go to bed. He was due to sit his finals in a few weeks but was feeling increasingly stressed and worried as the exams loomed nearer.

The more he revised, the less he seemed to retain. Even more worryingly when he sat past exam papers and timed himself against the clock his mind would go blank and a sense of dread would overtake him, meaning he forgot all he had revised. He would throw the exam papers onto the floor berating himself that he couldn't remember any answers. Yet once he calmed down he would be furious when he checked his notes and realised he had revised the right answers but was unable to recall them.

Milo had worked so hard over the last three years and didn't want to fall at the last hurdle, yet the harder he tried the more panic he felt. His housemates tried to tell him he was *'burning the candle at both ends'* but they didn't understand he had to graduate with top grades – anything else could not be tolerated.

His aim was to work for one of the top three accounting firms in the country and he knew they only accepted the best. This had been his goal since starting university and anything less would be seen as a failure. He wanted to enter the accounting profession as he had always liked numbers and believed it to be a safe career with good pay and pension.

He wondered about turning off the light and trying to get some sleep but instinctively knew that sleep would evade him. He often felt peace watching the sunrise, and his housemates would stagger downstairs groggy from their night's sleep but rarely looking surprised when they saw him staring out of the window with a coffee in his hands. Milo was constantly tired, and his face reflected it, etched with worry and dark shadows under his eyes.

Just recently he had started to feel a sense of desperation overtaking him like a dark cloud and had even started to wonder what the point of it all was. He could be consumed by these thoughts for days on end yet never really seemed to find an answer. Sighing he picked up his revision notes and started again.

Remember ... you've got this

Milo is suffering from burnout – a feeling of exhaustion created by becoming all consumed with revising. Like everything in life, there must be a balance between work and rest. Your body needs to take the time to recover and refuel.

Milo is in fear, which means hormones are being released which inhibit the logical part of his brain from working. When you obsess and worry you start to panic, and this means you are unable to recall facts and figures. Unable to take a step back and review the situation logically and objectively, you become obsessed and unable to feel hope or see clarity in a situation.

Milo has placed all his expectations in the 'I must work for XYZ accountants for me to be happy' basket. This is causing him mental anguish, especially when he thinks he may not achieve it. The worry of not being successful is affecting his present, and his mental health is suffering including his sleep. He is questioning his future and is unable to see other options apart from the fixed outcome he has set for himself.

However, if Milo can trust in himself and the bigger picture, his worry will dissipate if he can believe that whatever results he obtains means the right path will unfold. Knowing he is still lovable and worthy regardless of his results means he will increase feelings of self-belief and reduce his self-doubt.

Once Milo can realise that the right organisation will value his work ethic, tenacity and commitment then he can trust that whatever happens is the right thing for him. Maybe working for one of the top three accounting firms is not right for his personality? Entering a different accountancy firm may mean there is more chance of promotion and is a better environment for the type of person he is.

The best option for Milo is to go and speak to his tutor or lecturer who could reassure him. He could also research how to have a better sleep routine and take some exercise out in nature. Natural sunlight, water and sleep are all restorative along with being shown some help and support.

If Milo can be kinder to himself and allow himself to believe he is more than his results and be able to let go of his rigid expectations, then he will feel much better. Knowing his self-belief and self-worth is not attached to a job or exam results is critical.

TOPIC 7.1 I FEEL SO ANXIOUS, I DON'T THINK I AM ABLE TO SIT MY EXAMS

Sitting exams is a stressful time for many due to the pressure of passing and doing your best. The fear of failing affecting your future plans can understandably cause you to worry. However, if you *think* you are going to fail, then these negative thoughts trigger the release of hormones into your bloodstream which activate your fight and flight response, increasing anxious symptoms and stopping your logical thinking.

You can stop this from happening by changing your thoughts about your current situation to more positive, loving and compassionate thoughts. Once you can learn how to speak lovingly to yourself, your fear disappears.

Consider these two scenarios.

SIAN

Before her exam, Sian is sitting nervously rereading her notes, too upset to eat any breakfast. Wanting to achieve high marks she sees anything less as a failure. She thinks high marks will secure her a good job and is applying a lot of pressure on herself because of this belief. Sian has always achieved top grades and rarely fails at anything in her life. Her conditioned fear of failure is huge which causes great anxiety at times like this.

MO

Mo is laughing with his friends outside the exam hall. He had a good night's sleep as he went on a long walk the day before in the fresh air. He is looking forward to sitting his exam as he knows it is a way of showcasing his knowledge on the subject. He feels he has committed 100 per cent to his studies and could not have tried any harder. Mo also knows his future is not wholly reliant on exam results but is also dependent on his positive attitude, trust in the universe and a belief that he is an asset to any organisation.

Mo understands that fearful thinking creates symptoms called anxiety, and he understands the power of speaking positive kind words to himself and trusting everything will be okay, regardless of his exam results. While it is important to try your best in life, being able to let go of control and trust what is meant to be helps surrender your worries.

Repeating affirmations such as, *my best is enough* or *I can handle this* or *I know I will achieve the right grades for* me will help calm your fearful thoughts, meaning you access your thinking brain, recalling the data you need to pass your exams.

Passing exams may seem such a huge problem now, but in time you will realise it is just part of the university system.

SELF-ENQUIRY REFLECTION 7.1

. . . .

Not giving your personal power away to sitting exams is essential. Exam taking is simply part of university life and minimising the effect it can have on your emotions is important. These questions will help you work out how much power you are giving to the exams and results.

I have the courage to trust the outcome of my exam results.

1. On a scale of 0–10 (10 being the maximum), how worried am I about sitting exams?

2. What specifically am I worried about?

3. How much pressure am I applying to myself and how can I alleviate this pressure?

4. What do I think will happen if I get poor results?

5. How can I speak more lovingly to myself about the exam process?
   (*What would you advise a friend who was worried about their exam results?*)

LIFE LESSON

. . . .

It is highly likely that there will be times in your working life when you are tested, such as job interviews or promotions. Staying calm and centred through thinking positive and not allowing your fear to disturb your mindset is key to your future success and mental well-being.

TOPIC 7.2 I WANT TO GIVE UP AS I KNOW I AM GOING TO FAIL MY EXAMS

Wanting to give up as the exam period approaches is understandable and is often rooted in fear. Quitting is a common reaction when faced with pressure as it means you can escape the emotional pain you are feeling. If you are feeling this way, fear may have stopped your logical thinking and you have lost the ability to apply reasoned thinking. You are probably telling yourself you are going to fail so what's the point in continuing anyway. Be kind to yourself, you have done too well to give up now.

When you want to give up, ask yourself the following questions.

- Do I really want to give up or do I just want a rest?
- Am I really wanting to quit, or do I simply want to escape the emotional pain I am feeling?
- What were my goals when I started university?
- What am I hoping to gain at the end of my university experience and why is this important to me?
- If I quit, how will I feel when the exams are over?
- What are my options if I quit now?
- Is quitting the right decision really?
- If I knew I would pass my exams, would I still want to quit?

Some people quit as it seems the only option in the short term as it eases the burden and emotional pain, but in the long term they can regret their choice. However, giving yourself permission to quit can often relieve the pressure and helps you realise you don't really want to quit.

Taking the time to ask yourself the questions above may help you realise it was never about quitting, just a wish to escape the overwhelming emotions you are feeling which is completely understandable. When you are feeling overwhelmed, receiving psychological support is key to help reassure you that you can pass your exams. Your lecturer or tutor will appreciate how you feel and can provide words of encouragement and reassurance help you continue your journey.

Be kind and compassionate with yourself. Look at how far you have come. Remember the university experience is one of learning about yourself, your strengths and the areas you need to personally develop. Maybe learning to be gentle with yourself and reaching out for help are two areas you need to learn right now?

Ask yourself what is the most empowering decision I can make right now?

SELF-ENQUIRY REFLECTION 7.2

....

Wanting to give up is a normal human reaction and sometimes letting go of something is the right choice. However, if wanting to give up is rooted in fear then it is sensible to talk to someone else about your decision to ensure it is made for the right reasons.

I have the courage to investigate why I want to give up.

1. On a scale of 0–10 (10 being the maximum), how much do I want to give up?

2. What are my reasons for wanting to give up?

3. What would giving up give me right now?

4. What would giving up give me long term?

5. What would not giving up give me long term?

LIFE LESSON

....

There will be times in your life when you want to give up on something. It may be a job, relationship, study or a project of some kind. It is important to know the real reasons underlying why you want to quit and talk it through with someone who can help you. Sometimes we do need to let go of something, yet this is very different from giving up.

TOPIC 7.3 I AM NOT VERY GOOD AT REVISING AS I GET DISTRACTED

It is understandable you get distracted when revising as it is certainly not the most fun activity in the world. However, revision is part of the university process and committing to your revision will help you feel more in control of securing a good result.

Practical tips for minimising distractions

- Set yourself a schedule of what you need to revise and allocate time to each task. Reward yourself with a distraction break when you have finished each task.
- Have distraction breaks where you can check your phone, message your friend or scroll on social media.
- Ensure you have refreshments handy so you don't have to stop which may encourage distractions.
- Remove distractions such as your mobile phone or if you have it near you, turn off notifications and place it face down so you cannot see anything pop onto the screen.
- Tell people to not disturb you.
- Link your revision to your long-term goals – what is this act of revising going to help you achieve? Be aware that if you distract, it may sabotage your goals.
- Have a schedule and mark off your tasks so you can see how much progress you are making.
- Make a choice – will you allow yourself to get distracted or not?

Revising for exams can be a test of determination and tenacity. Committing 100 per cent to the life choice of studying at university means allocating your energy and time to ensure you revise to the best of your ability.

Being able to look back and say you committed 100 per cent to your revision and that you are proud of what you achieved is a great position to be in. It is difficult to live the rest of your life knowing you did not try your best, so take this time to commit to the best you are able to do. However, also be mindful of other priorities in your life. You may need to delegate tasks to other people so that you can revise as much as possible.

It is also important to learn to balance revision time with fun activities, so you do not suffer from revision burnout. Be gentle with yourself and listen to your body to help maximise your revision opportunities. If your brain is too tired, it will be harder to revise, and you may need to rest. You may prefer revising at times when others are asleep for example. It is your revision schedule, so own it.

SELF-ENQUIRY REFLECTION 7.3

....

Revision is one of life's activities which you wouldn't naturally choose to do; however, it is usually needed to pass exams. Being disciplined with yourself will help you commit to the task at hand. These questions will help you discern how you can take responsibility to ensure you do this.

I have the courage to commit to my revision.

1. On a scale of 0–10 (10 being the maximum), how much am I struggling to commit to my revision?

2. If I was committing 10 out of 10 to my revision, what would I be doing differently?

3. What is stopping me from taking these actions?

4. If I committed to my revision, what would be the benefit to me, my mental health and my future?

5. How can I balance my revision with rest and the other priorities in my life?

LIFE LESSON

....

Throughout your life there will be times when it will become challenging and committing 100 per cent to an outcome is essential. Success usually comes from tenacity and not giving up. Remembering why you started something in the first place will help you continue. Be proud of your self-motivation and know this creates a more empowered you. However, also be aware of when you need to rest and have a break.

TOPIC 7.4 I AM TIRED OF REVISING FOR MY EXAMS, BUT HAVE I DONE ENOUGH?

Revising for exams can be a monumental task which few people enjoy, yet accepting revision is part of the university experience and knowing you probably won't ever have to do it again once you have finished can alleviate some of your pain. Many students think they have not revised enough before they sit exams.

Even though you may have spent a lot of time revising, nerves can still take over as the day of the exam approaches. However, if you have attended lectures, kept up with your coursework and followed a revision plan, you have done all you can to succeed. Your revision is simply a consolidation of your knowledge and sitting the exam is showcasing this.

It is important you realise you are not in full control of exam results and can only influence them. For example, you may get some tricky or unexpected questions which you did not expect. Therefore, trust you have tried your best and accept that your best really is good enough, then let go of the worry. If you have perfectionist tendencies, you may believe you have not done enough but it is essential you feel proud of all you have achieved.

Ensure your self-worth is not connected to your exam results. This means you only believe you are good enough if you get outstanding results. This is an unhealthy viewpoint to have as it means your self-worth is dependent on external validation. Understand you are worthy simply for being you and the positive difference you make to this world.

Talk kindly to yourself and reassure yourself that you are being brave in choosing to sit your exams. Not everyone manages to get this far, and you need to congratulate yourself for doing so well, regardless of your results.

Try not to compare yourself to others with regards to your revision schedule. People retain knowledge in different ways and comparing yourself to another can lead to worry. Your circumstances in life may mean that you are unable to revise the same amount as your friends. Know you are doing your best and managing the best you can under the circumstances. Trust that whatever happens, you can handle it!

SELF-ENQUIRY REFLECTION 7.4

....

Most students think they have not revised enough, however, think logically, not emotionally, about the situation. Could you really do anymore? If so, then keep going, taking into account how much energy you have left. However, if you truly believe you have done enough, then allow yourself some downtime.

I have the courage to trust in the revision I have completed.

1. On a scale of 0–10, (10 being the maximum) how tired am I of revising for my exams?

2. How adequate is the revision I have completed?

3. How much more revision do I think I can do?

4. What difference do I think this will make?

5. What kind words can I say to myself about the revision I have completed?

LIFE LESSON

....

Be appreciative of the effort you have committed to your revision. You will have balanced it with other demands in your life so well done. Be kind to yourself and be your own best friend. Reassure yourself that your best is good enough and you are a success because you tried.

TOPIC 7.5 I AM WORRIED I WILL FORGET EVERYTHING WHEN I SIT MY EXAMS

Many students worry they will struggle to remember their revision when they sit their exam. This is the power of fear – it stops your logical brain from working. The more thoughts you have about failing, the more anxious you can feel, which affects the recall of the facts and figures you need.

However, the good news is this temporary amnesia is completely avoidable. Embracing the ideas below will ensure you create the right mindset to remember everything you need to gain outstanding results.

1. Ensure you are sleeping as well as you can. This may mean avoiding alcohol and any other form of stimulants leading up to the exams.
2. Surround yourself with positivity – this means avoiding the news or any people who are draining and negative – you don't want your positive vibes being sucked out of you.
3. Ensure you are eating healthily and drinking plenty of water – this ensures the energy flows around your body, allowing conscious thinking.
4. Don't talk about possible exam content before you enter the exam hall as this may trigger your fears.
5. Repeat calming affirmations such as *I can handle it*, or *I achieve the results I want* or *I can do this*. The silent repetition of these affirmations will help calm your fearful brain meaning you access your logical brain.
6. Look forward to the day when exams are over, and you are finally free from revision and studying.
7. Remind yourself that whatever happens, you will handle it and you are a success for committing to university life.
8. Trust there is a bigger picture to your life, and you are more than your exam results. Whatever results you get, will be the right results for your journey in life.
9. Be proud of how far you have come and all the work you have completed to get yourself to sit the exam. Your tenacity will be rewarded.
10. Keep breathing! Take three deep breaths in and exhale slowly before you turn the exam paper over and remind yourself, *I can do this*.
11. After the exam do not berate yourself when you hear others talk about what they wrote. Remember it is only their perception, they are not examiners.
12. Celebrate the completion of the exam and look forward to fun with your friends, enjoying your own company or spending time with loved ones.

Taking exams is one short chapter in your life and it will pass; fun times will come.

SELF-ENQUIRY REFLECTION 7.5

....

Thoughts regarding failing to remember your revision is simply fear taking over. Engage a more powerful voice and tell your fear that you will succeed. Remember, you are good enough and will achieve the right results for you and your journey.

I have the courage to stay calm while sitting my exams.

1. On a scale of 0–10 (10 being the maximum), how worried am I that I may forget everything I have learned?

2. What three techniques above can I use to keep calm?

3. When have I previously sat exams and remembered the answers?

4. How can I be kinder to myself about this situation?

5. What would I say to someone else who has revised the amount I have?

LIFE LESSON

....

Not allowing the emotion of fear to overwhelm you ensures your life is enjoyable. Of course, you will have fears in your life, but learning to overcome them means you become more confident as you build a healthy trust in knowing you can handle everything which comes your way.

TOPIC 7.6 I'VE FAILED TO GET THE EXAM RESULTS I WANTED

You may be feeling disappointed, even worried, that you have not achieved the exam results you wanted. Whatever stage of the university process you are at, this can mean you start doubting yourself, perhaps even thinking you are not clever enough or a failure.

This of course is untrue; exams are a test of your understanding of a subject with the ability to memorise and convey facts and data within a specified framework. This is just one aspect of university life and some people do struggle to share everything they have learned in a time-pressured environment. You have many other skills and attributes which prove you are worthy to attend university and pass your course.

The first step in managing disappointing grades is to accept the way you feel is okay and allow yourself to grieve. This is a loss, so take the time to accept this, ensuring you are kind and compassionate with yourself.

Next, focus on the future, not the past – you tried your best, committed as much as you could and now it is time to let the past go and focus on your future. However, it is important to learn from the experience and obtaining feedback is a great way to do this. If you understand which areas you performed well in and your lecturer highlights improvement areas this will help support your progression and achievement.

You may also want to ask yourself a tough question – how could I have taken responsibility to obtain better marks? If you can admit where you can improve this is a big step to future success.

Remember your exam results are just one aspect of your university experience so do not allow your self-worth to be dependent on your results. These results may seem like a huge deal to you now, but it is just one chapter of your life. You have many more exciting chapters to live so have the self-belief that you can and will excel. Being emotionally resilient means handling situations positively and bouncing back from adversity.

Reach out to those who can offer you words of comfort and advice, whether that be your favourite lecturer, a family member or friend. In time your disappointment will dissipate, and you can move on, knowing you were good enough all along.

SELF-ENQUIRY REFLECTION 7.6

. . . .

Regardless of the outcome, not giving your power away to a set of exam results is important. Stay logical, not emotional about them. There is always something to learn in life, so reflect on where you can improve and let the rest go.

I have the courage to learn from this experience.

1. On a scale of 0–10 (10 being the maximum), how disappointed am I regarding my exam results?

2. How can I talk kindly to myself about my results, regardless of the outcome?

3. What can I learn from this situation?

4. What other skills and traits do I have which I am proud of?

5. Who can I speak to who can help me deal with this situation?

LIFE LESSON

. . . .

Disappointment can feel painful, but it is a necessary feeling to experience. You may be so disappointed that you cry, and this is okay. This reaction is simply acknowledging a loss. When you have expressed the emotion, you will rise again. Being able to handle challenging life experiences is called resilience and is a great skill to possess.

TOPIC 7.7 I WANT TO LEAVE UNIVERSITY WITH A FIRST-CLASS HONOURS DEGREE

You may put a lot of pressure on yourself to obtain a first in your studies. While having a goal to aim for is commendable, if it is causing you stress, anxiety and worry then it's too much of a high price to pay. Your grades are simply one part of your university experience, and your future career is not solely dependent on obtaining a first.

University is about discovering you, the type of person you are, and the type of person you want to be, in effect what makes you tick. While the academic side of university is important, developing your self-awareness, self-belief and self-trust is far more important than a set of grades.

University is a time to discover.

- What difference do you want to make in the world?
- How would you want to be described by another?
- What life experiences do you want to enjoy?
- What life experiences do you want to avoid?
- What makes you happy and sad?
- What are you good at and what aspects of yourself do you want to change?
- What excites you and makes you passionate about life?
- What type of people do you want to be surrounded by?
- How can you be free from worry?

Many students see a first-class honours result as the ultimate success and as a testament to their hard work, which of course it can be. However, leaving university as a more self-aware, confident individual than when you started means you have matured and developed as a person, and will therefore be an asset to any organisation.

If you receive a lower mark than you would have liked but have increased your confidence and self-belief in addition to making some great friends and created life-changing memories, then this has been a valuable university experience. Some employers prefer a fully rounded individual who can express themselves, believe in their abilities and know they are an asset to the organisation more than simply a first-class academic result.

So, take the pressure off yourself, be reassured you are enough regardless of the grade you receive. Invest some time and energy into finding out more about yourself and the difference you want to make in this world. You are here for a reason and the exciting adventure is finding out what this is.

SELF-ENQUIRY REFLECTION 7.7

There can be social pressure to achieve high marks and while it is commendable to try your best, realising this is not the only goal of university can help put your grades in perspective. Taking the pressure off yourself and identifying how else university success can be defined is a mature way to view the situation.

I have the courage to take the pressure off myself.

1. On a scale of 0–10 (10 being the maximum), how much am I pressurising myself to achieve a first-class grade?

2. What are my reasons for wanting this result?

3. How is this expectation making me feel?

4. What story am I telling myself if I don't get this grade?

5. How can I reframe this story to relieve the pressure I am feeling?

LIFE LESSON

You may have been conditioned to strive for top marks in your studies. However, the university experience is different as it is not only about achieving grades but also about personal and professional development. Self-awareness is a great skill to have in life to achieve happiness both personally and professionally.

TOPIC 7.8 IF I DON'T GET GOOD GRADES, I AM SCARED I WON'T GET A JOB

....

Many students fear that if they fail to get good grades, they will not get the job of their dreams. While some organisations do have certain entry-level requirements, there are plenty of other companies which value intrinsic skills such as confidence and critical thinking rather than just a university grade. Therefore, reassure yourself that whatever grades you achieve, you will be the right fit with an organisation which suits you.

Remember that applying for graduate schemes or jobs is a two-way process. Yes, you are being interviewed by the organisation; however, take the time to discern if the organisation suits the type of person, you are. Satisfy yourself that you and the organisation are a good match, akin to entering a relationship. You may feel pressurised to take the first job offered to you, but if you are not buzzing with excitement, it may not be the right choice. Talk to someone you trust to help you decide.

Many organisations are not overly focused on you having a certain grade as they conduct their own internal assessment procedures to make sure you are a good fit. Therefore, being confident in your abilities means you can complete their assessment days and showcase what an asset you will be to them.

Some organisations still encourage you to apply for their schemes, even if you have just missed out on a certain grade, so it is always worth contacting the company and asking if it is worth you apply.

If your grades are low and you are unsure of what job you would like, you may decide you want to start your own business. If you are passionate about a product or service or see a gap in a market, consider being your own boss. There is plenty of support in setting up your own business, and running your own company is one of the most exciting journeys to travel.

Many graduates leave university not really knowing what they want to do, and this is okay. Volunteering or completing an internship can also be a great way to gain experience and identify the type of work you want to do and the difference you want to make in the world.

Although not getting the grades you want can feel disappointing, your strength lies in being able to handle disappointments and still taking action to live the life you want to live.

SELF-ENQUIRY REFLECTION 7.8

Coping with all that happens in your life with a positive attitude means you will always handle setbacks. Knowing you will have a successful life regardless of your grades will help calm your anxieties.

I have the courage to allow my future to unfold.

1. On a scale of 0–10 (10 being the maximum), how much do I believe I will struggle to find a successful job if I receive low grades?

2. What evidence do I have which is making me believe this?

3. What would I tell a friend to contradict this evidence?

4. What other options would I have if I don't get the grades I want?

5. How can I reassure myself or who can I speak to reassure me that everything will work out for the best?

LIFE LESSON

Being adaptable in life is key to your happiness. Sometimes you fail to get what you think you want, yet these obstacles are a cosmic gift from the universe. Being open to plans B, C and D and being flexible enough to change your goals is a great way to enjoy life. Maintaining a positive attitude is key when you face disappointment; however, this also means you allow yourself to feel whatever your feel.

CHAPTER 8
TRANSITIONING INTO ADULTHOOD

. . . .

Adulthood is like the vet, and we're all the dogs that were excited for the car ride until we found out where we were going.

Author unknown

SCENARIO

. . . .

Autumn was usually Dihanna's favourite time of the year as she loved to walk in the woods observing the beautiful colours of the leaves which had fallen from the trees. Yet today, she didn't see any of this as she was struggling to cope with the searing pain in her heart. Even though walking in solitude was one of her favourite things to do when she felt upset, she was struggling to breathe as the tears poured down her face.

She had tried calling her mum with no answer, but Dihanna took some solace in knowing what her mum would say when she told her how she was feeling today. Her mum was a spiritual psychologist and had taught her to fully walk into feeling the pain, surrender to the universe and trust that healing and spiritual insights would come in time.

While this way of thinking had been hard for Dihanna to accept as she was growing up as it was very different from how her friends were raised, she now fully understood the importance of being able to live life spiritually. It didn't mean she was immune to challenging life events, in fact sometimes it felt the opposite, but it did mean that she took as much responsibility as she could to learn what her soul was needing to learn from the experience and therefore had to allow herself to be directed by her heart.

Yet two weeks ago was a particularly hard soul lesson when she found out her boyfriend of six months, Cameron, had slept with his ex when he had visited home for the weekend. Even though he had sat Dihanna down and explained the situation as soon as he returned to university, the physical and emotional pain she had felt was excruciating. The pain had lessened a little in the last couple of days, but she would have moments like now where it would come flooding back. Her mum had explained it was simply her heart clearing the emotional energy of grief which was much needed for her to find peace in the long term and with time it would pass, yet it had to be experienced not fought against.

Not caring if anyone saw her tears, she stayed focused on her breathing to regain some self-control and composure. She knew the importance of calming her emotional self as she needed to think logically when she met Cameron in an hour's time.

Dihanna had spent the last week reclaiming her power. Sure, she had spent some time crying to her best friend who had called Cam all sorts of names. Although this had helped at the time, Dihanna knew it wasn't that easy to stop feeling what she felt for him. However, she did know she had to take responsibility for herself so had asked Cameron to leave her alone for two weeks to give her some time to heal and think. She had spent the time having a session of reiki healing to help her emotionally and had journaled about how she felt. Her mum's friend was an astrologer, so she had booked a consultation with her and had been shown what the universe was wanting her to learn from this situation.

Dihanna knew she needed to have an honest conversation with Cameron which would not be pleasant, and she didn't know what he would say, yet she did know she would feel better simply by speaking her truth and having the conversation. If truth be told, the red flags had been there when she first met Cam, but she had chosen not to see them, carried away by the feeling of being wanted and loved by another. She didn't know what the outcome would be from their conversation today but what she did know was she could handle the outcome, whatever it was.

....

TRANSITIONING INTO ADULTHOOD

Remember ... you've got this

The more you embrace adulthood the more life experiences you will have. Some of these experiences will be amazing and joyful and some may cause you pain and upset, especially in matters of the heart.

However, whatever happens to you can be viewed as a life experience which will help to empower you. It does this by teaching you how strong and resilient you really are to cope with challenging times. Having a tool bag of strategies and techniques to help handle challenging life experiences throughout adulthood is important. These techniques include physical such as exercising, psychological which includes journalling how you feel and asking for help and spiritual interventions which help you understand the bigger picture at play.

Adulthood can be an emotionally painful time but through this, you must not be afraid of feeling all your emotions which highlight where you can take responsibility (action) to make your life as peaceful as you can. Making decisions and not being fearful of any outcome means you can handle anything which happens to you, and this is how you become truly confident and authentically yourself.

It is easy to get overwhelmed by your emotions at times and, just like a child, want to rush to another to make everything okay for you. However, this is often not the most empowering thing to do as you can become dependent on another to make you feel better. Then if something happens to this person you can feel alone, like a lost child, which can trigger feelings of abandonment leading to anxiety symptoms. Adulthood is realising you can stand alone yet knowing when to ask another for support.

Adulthood can also challenge many ways of thinking you have been taught as a child and this can be painful. You may realise you have not been taught the most empowering ways to think and act; however, this is no criticism of those who have raised you, they could only teach you the ways they have been taught to think and cope.

Being an adult means exploring how you want to think, feel and behave in ways which may differ from those around you. As an adult, you have the right to challenge others, even those who you may see as having authority over you. Learning positive ways to think, feel and behave and knowing you can handle adversity means you will succeed in life both personally and professionally.

TOPIC 8.1 EMBRACE CHANGE

· ·

Resisting change is natural, as change pushes you out of the familiar into the unknown. The unknown is scary as it can produce feelings you have not felt before which can make you feel uncomfortable. It is usual to have comfort zones; this comfort zone is what feels familiar to you, helps you feel safe and reassured as you know what is going to happen and therefore how you will feel.

Examples of comfort zones are:

- your daily habits and routines;
- your day-to-day activities – work, education, meals, hobbies, interests sleep;
- people in your life – how they behave towards you and vice versa.

> ### EXAMPLE
>
> Take a moment to reflect on your morning routine. Do you wake up, reach for your phone, and start scrolling on social media? Before you know it, have 20 minutes disappeared without you even realising it? This is an example of a comfort zone – *a programmed set of behaviours (habits) where you automatically behave in the same way, often without much conscious thought.*
>
> What other familiar comfort zones do you have during the day and how do they make you feel – joyful and free or secure and in control?

While comfort zones can be great as they provide structure and make you feel in control, they can also hold you back from authentically living and experiencing new opportunities.

Leaving home to attend university probably pushed you out of your comfort zone into a strange environment which might have made you feel unsafe and scared. You may have started to worry and imagined awful scenarios. The more you think about bad things happening to you, the more you worry and before you know it, you are stuck in a cycle of negative thinking and experiencing uncomfortable physiological symptoms due to the release of hormones into your bloodstream. Many people refer to this as anxiety and it feels very real.

To avoid feeling this way, some people resist making changes and the natural reaction is to stop what you are considering doing and retreat into safety meaning you stay stuck in your comfort zone.

> ### WARNING * WARNING * WARNING * WARNING
>
> Some people fear handling the unknown, so they stay in their comfort zone, which means they rarely take risks, never learning they can handle

the unknown. The familiarity makes them feel safe, yet this safety doesn't give them the excitement and the fulfilment they deserve. Who do you know who has lived in their comfort zone all their life, rarely taking creative risks to live a more expansive life?

It is important that you become comfortable using your courage to take action to push yourself out of your comfort zone and not let your fear of the unknown hold you back. This then allows the anxious symptoms to disappear as you realise you can handle the unknown.

SELF-ENQUIRY REFLECTION 8.1

A great psychological strategy to use to help you move out of your comfort zone is to know what scares you about the unknown and then ask yourself, can I handle these fears? Being able to embrace change will ensure you live a rich and fulfilled life.

I have the courage to embrace change.

1. On a scale of 0–10 (10 being the maximum), how comfortable am I choosing to leave the familiar and move out of my comfort zone?

2. On a scale of 0–10 (10 being the maximum), how comfortable am I being pushed out of my comfort zone?

3. What fears may be stopping me from making changes or handling changes which have been forced upon me?

4. What have I realised about myself and what comfort zones am I in?

5. How can I encourage myself to embrace change more?

LIFE LESSON

Moving out of your comfort zone is how you learn to embrace change, knowing you can handle the unknown. It is a sign of maturity as you are displaying inner strength and confidence. When you start to feel as though you are resisting changes, ask yourself, what am I fearing, take action to overcome your fears and reassure yourself you can handle whatever happens.

TOPIC 8.2 SPEAK YOUR TRUTH

Speaking your truth means you have the confidence to say what you want to say, even in emotional situations. Of course, there may be times when speaking your truth may upset another person, yet courage is not allowing this fear to stop you. If you speak your truth from a place of love, compassion and respect for yourself and the other person, then you are being authentic.

The truth you speak is simply based on the way you see the world. Others can have a different truth based on how they see the world. This difference in perception means you may disagree with others yet can still remain compassionate and loving towards them.

Owning your truth means you say what you want to say lovingly while accepting that others may react in a way which makes you feel uncomfortable. Being able to disagree yet stay in harmony with the other person is a sign of maturity.

If someone says you have made them angry or upset, then reassure yourself that it wasn't your intention to be cruel, but you had to be true to yourself. Remember you do not have the power to make another person feel a certain way – if what you have said has triggered something in them, their self-awareness can help them to explore this. Let them take responsibility for their own feelings, it is not your responsibility to carry their feelings anymore.

Of course, there will be times when speaking your truth will provoke an argument and you may get triggered by someone's heightened emotions. This is not a time to berate yourself if you do lose your composure, but you may need to apologise and listen to their view of the situation. The person you are disagreeing with may not have the same self-awareness to do this so be aware that you may still not achieve harmony.

It is important to realise that your truth is only your opinion, and the other person does not have to agree with you. In fact, others disagreeing with your opinion can often be a good thing as it helps you take a step back and ask if your perception is valid or if your opinion needs changing in any way.

The more you practice speaking your truth with love, the easier it becomes to handle others' reactions as you know you are not intentionally causing them pain. Of course, if you speak your truth then others may want to speak their truth with you. This can often be painful, hearing another's opinions on a subject, especially if their opinions are about you in some way. It is understandable you may get emotionally triggered which means you react defensively. While this can feel uncomfortable, it can be an opportunity for you to later reflect on what made you defensive. Perhaps the person was giving you good feedback which you may have needed to hear to help you discern if a behaviour change is needed. Of course, you may choose not to agree with their feedback, in which case you can let it go and move on.

SELF-ENQUIRY REFLECTION 8.2

....

If you speak your truth with love then no matter how the other person reacts, you know your intentions were positive and you meant no harm. You cannot control how another person will react and being able to handle uncomfortable situations resulting from speaking your truth means you are a confident individual.

I have the courage to speak my truth with love.

1. On a scale of 0–10 (10 being the maximum), how comfortable am I speaking my truth with love?

2. How do I resist speaking my truth?

3. What am I scared of happening if I speak my truth?

4. What can I tell myself, so I have the confidence to speak my truth?

5. What is the truth I need to speak to someone now?

LIFE LESSON

....

Your truth can change as your perception changes. Life is about evolving as a human and learning new things about yourself, others and life in general. Being able to admit; this is my truth based on what I know now is a sign of maturity and always means you can change your mind in the future.

TOPIC 8.3 BE COMFORTABLE BEING DISLIKED

....

It is common to be a people-pleaser which means you put others' needs first at the risk of not pleasing yourself. You may do this as you do not like the feeling of upsetting others, either because you don't want to see the other person in emotional pain, or you do not want to risk facing their anger, sulking or disapproval.

We become a people-pleaser based on our past. As a child, someone important to you may have withdrawn their love and attention simply because you didn't behave in the way they wanted or expected you to. This inconsistency hurts on a physical level, as it makes you feel scared, abandoned and alone. To avoid feeling this pain as an adult, you may behave in a way to ensure people approve of you, thinking they may not withdraw their love, hence we become a people-pleaser.

However, people-pleasing can affect your well-being as you spend your time and energy meeting another's needs and not meeting your own. While it is important to be mindful of others and not intentionally cause them harm, it is necessary for you to learn to meet your own needs – whether these are physical, emotional, spiritual or mental. It is your responsibility to prioritise meeting your needs to help you build your inner strength, confidence and self-worth and inner-child healing is an effective way to help you achieve this.

When you decide you want to stop being a people-pleaser and start to prioritise your needs, others around you may be displeased with you because you are not prioritising them. However, it is important to be surrounded by people who care for your happiness and want the best for you. While it can be a painful realisation that those around you may not want this for you, it is better to know this than be in a painful illusion of being surrounded by selfish people, even if these people are family.

When you start to assert your needs either at home, university or work, it may trigger an emotional reaction in others. The other person may try and blame you for making them feel a certain way. However, you do not have the power to make another feel a certain way; it is how they are choosing to react. They have probably been emotionally triggered in some way. While it is important not to intentionally hurt another, a balance must be made of prioritising your own well-being while not causing another unnecessary pain.

The more comfortable you are being disliked, realising that not everyone will like you, the more willing and able you are to prioritise your needs.

SELF-ENQUIRY REFLECTION 8.3

Some people don't want to be disliked as they think it means they are mean or even unlovable. However, there is nothing mean about meeting your own needs to ensure your well-being is a priority. In fact, when you are comfortable meeting your own needs, you are more willing and able to meet another's.

I have the courage to be disliked.

1. On a scale of 0–10 (10 being the maximum), how comfortable am I being disliked?

2. What concerns me about being disliked and which is more important to me – being liked or protecting my well-being?

3. How may I be people-pleasing right now?

4. How can I stop people-pleasing and meet my own needs?

5. How can I reframe being disliked by others?

LIFE LESSON

Others may dislike you when you start to assert yourself because you are thinking differently or behaving in a way which they do not agree with which may cause them pain. The easiest reaction for them is to not like you instead of reflecting on themselves. However, learning how to like and love yourself is one of most important soul lessons in life.

TOPIC 8.4 QUESTION HOW YOU HAVE BEEN TAUGHT TO THINK

From an early age, you are taught what to think by those around you – this includes your caregivers, educators, friends, social media, television programmes, your religious upbringing and society in general. The way you have been trained to think results in a *conditioned belief system*. Because of this conditioning, you may not have a healthy belief system which will affect your well-being and life choices.

You will have many beliefs about many things. Some include:

- what you can achieve – your potential regarding your career;
- your personality – whether you are attractive, funny or kind;
- your body image, sexuality and relationship preferences;
- how you and others should behave in relationships;
- if the world is safe or scary;
- whether you can trust yourself or others;
- love, intimacy and sex;
- politics, religion and current affairs.

As you are mature into an independent thinker, those around you may have such strong beliefs about a certain subject and believe their way of thinking is right. They may not like you thinking differently to them and dislike you for making certain life choices. This can be painful, especially when it is your family.

An example of a strong belief system is a man who became a doctor simply because his own father who was also a doctor wanted him to follow in the family footsteps. Strongly believing his own son should keep the family tradition, he expects his son to even though his son doesn't want to. He rejects the son because the son wants to follow his passion of being an activist for those less fortunate than himself.

Belief systems can affect daily life, especially relationships.

EXAMPLE

Lilly watches the evening news as she eats her evening meal. If you asked Lily why she does that, she would explain it is a way of finding out what is happening in the world. When she later reflects, Lily realises she does it because as a child she watched her parents watch the news as they ate their evening meal. It is Lily's belief that the news is an accurate representation of what is happening in the world, and it is what you do.

Luke doesn't watch the news on the television as his mum taught him that the negative content can provoke an internal response of fear due to the doom and gloom it shares. She suggested Luke research if the news is an accurate representation of what is happening in the world, and it is Luke's belief that the news can be a misrepresentation and should be treated with caution.

> If Lily and Luke started dating, there could be a difference in opinions due to different belief systems which may lead to arguments. However, if both parties are open to exploring each other's views, then the relationship could work.

In any relationship, being able to question your own beliefs and being open to hearing another's beliefs is a sign of maturity. Simply asking why you believe something to be true is an easy way to interrogate your belief system. Being willing to adapt your thinking is a sign of maturity, shows a high level of self-awareness and is a marketable skill.

SELF-ENQUIRY REFLECTION 8.4

Your belief system is developed by your early environment. Sadly, the way you think (your belief system) may not bring you happiness, yet you can change the way you think and develop a healthy set of new beliefs which feels right for you. Being able to question why you think the way you do is an act of self-awareness and essential in life.

I have the courage to reflect on the way I think.

1. On a scale of 0–10 (10 being the maximum), how willing am I to consider my belief system may not be healthy?
2. What would be the benefit of challenging the way I think (belief system) about certain subjects?
3. Why do I think some people are not open to having their viewpoint challenged?
4. What beliefs about myself do I have which may be holding me back in life or making me feel unhappy? (ie, *I'm not enough, unlovable or unintelligent*)
5. How can I start to change any unhealthy beliefs I hold?

LIFE LESSON

Self-awareness is when you reflect on why you think and behave the way you do. You have been taught to think and behave the way you do since you were small. Questioning your belief system and choosing more empowering ways to think can help you live a more authentic life, making life choices which are healthy for you.

TOPIC 8.5 POSITIVELY CHALLENGE PERCEIVED AUTHORITY

As you live your life you may perceive others as having authority over you and you have to do as you are told. In school, for example, you may have viewed your teacher as having authority over you and may have feared them. Appreciate now you are older, you are your own authority and while you can respect authority where warranted, you should not fear it.

To be able to positively challenge others no matter what role they play in your life, helps you build self-confidence. For example, you may view your parents as having authority and control over you, but is this true? They play the role of your parent, yet as an adult you are free to make your own choices in life, unless of course you are reliant on them for something. Sometimes what you want may be different from those around you but not fearing others' reactions is important for your psychological development and happiness.

You may not like challenging authority due to fears of:

- getting into trouble or being told off;
- being disapproved of, criticised or facing conflict;
- being seen as awkward or being told you are argumentative;
- being rejected or abandoned.

It is understandable that you may avoid challenging authority to avoid experiencing any of the above, however, being able to positively challenge authority and handle the consequences means you are maturing in a healthy way. Sometimes those in perceived authority may not like you challenging them, so it is important to challenge in a positive, constructive way. Remember challenging authority simply means you want to gain clarity, share your opinions or seek compromise.

EXAMPLE

If you seek medical advice and are unhappy with the diagnosis you have been given you may want to ask for a second opinion or challenge what you have been told. You may fear upsetting the person in authority, yet it may be essential in ensuring you are given the right information. It is okay to disagree with anybody, no matter what role they play in your life.

Knowing you have a right to seek further information or even say, I disagree or let's agree to disagree can be empowering. It is impossible for everyone to agree on everything as it is simply one's own perception and not the truth.

Being able to challenge another in a positive pro-active way means you are displaying assertiveness. Being assertive is a healthy sign of confidence. Even if others do not like you being assertive, it does not mean you stop doing it. Being able to handle the feelings of discomfort and disapproval, even if the authority figure does not like being challenged is also a sign of assertiveness.

SELF-ENQUIRY REFLECTION 8.5

....

Knowing you have a right to challenge authority, allows you to lose any perceived fears of doing so. Challenging in a positive, polite and respectful way means no matter how the other person reacts, you had a right to do so, and their reaction is their fear being acted out, not yours.

I have the courage to challenge perceived authority.

1. On a scale of 0–10 (10 being the maximum), how comfortable am I challenging perceived authority?

2. Who do I identify as a perceived authority?
   (*ie, parents, older family members, lecturers, doctor, consultants, police, government*)

3. What are my fears challenging perceived authority?

4. On a scale of 0–10 (10 being the maximum), how much do I feel I have a right to challenge perceived authority?

5. How can I challenge those around me in a positive, constructive way which makes me feel comfortable?

LIFE LESSON

....

Being comfortable challenging authority means you are not afraid of asserting yourself. Asserting yourself means you own what you say and deliver your message in a positive and empowering way. Often challenging authority can be helpful for the other person too as it allows them to possibly open their mind to alternative views.

TOPIC 8.6 HAVE HONEST CONVERSATIONS

· ·

Healthy relationships involve honest conversations, no matter how uncomfortable these conversations may be. In any relationship, you can have disagreements as no two people will think the same on every subject. However, being able to resolve disagreements in a mature adult way through communicating honestly and openly is key to bringing harmony.

You can resolve difficult situations by first admitting there is a problem and being willing to talk openly and honestly about it. This means you are transparent about how you feel without fear of retribution. Having an emotional conversation can be hard because you may not know how the other person is going to react and this may scare you, making you feel out of control. However, knowing you can handle any reaction is a sign of confidence.

Of course, you do not have to have an honest conversation to resolve a problem but ask yourself will anything change if the issue is not addressed. In fact, the problem may worsen so consider if you would rather live in a state of denial and pretence, rather than work together as a team to resolve things.

Before you have the honest conversation, answer the following questions:

- what is the issue which needs resolving?
- how am I responsible for this situation occurring?
- how is the other person responsible for the situation occurring?
- what would be the benefits of having an honest conversation?
- what would happen if we don't have the honest conversation?

Being willing to take responsibility for what has occurred means admitting what you may or may not have done to co-create the problem. This then puts you in a position of power as you are not afraid to admit you may have been wrong in some way and allows the other person to do the same, meaning true intimacy and respect develops. However, be aware that some people are unable to take responsibility, and you may have to accept this, but be mindful of the type of person you are dealing with.

When you have an honest conversation, remember you both may have different perceptions of how the situation has occurred: you do not have to agree but can still acknowledge each others' perception. Identifying a plan of action together for how the situation can be resolved is the final part in restoring harmony.

SELF-ENQUIRY REFLECTION 8.6

....

Having the courage to have an honest conversation means situations have a better chance of being resolved as issues are not ignored. While honest conversations can be uncomfortable conversations, they can lead to harmony, trust, intimacy and respect building between two people.

I have the courage to have an honest conversation.

1. On a scale of 0–10 (10 being the maximum), how comfortable am I in having honest conversations?

2. What do I like and dislike about having an honest conversation?

3. Who do I need to have an honest conversation with and what is the desired outcome I would like?

4. How can I take responsibility for the situation occurring?

5. How likely is it the other person can take responsibility for the situation occurring?

LIFE LESSON

....

Being able to have an honest conversation means you are not scared of facing reality and willing to resolve issues. Not being afraid of feeling uncomfortable while talking about emotional situations may help to resolve any difficulties and is a sign of maturity. Whether the other person is a child, parent, partner or work associate, being able to reach an agreed way forward is essential to help the situation resolve.

TOPIC 8.7 BALANCE GIVING AND RECEIVING HELP

You will meet people in your life who will benefit greatly from your time, love, energy and support. Being able to help others through challenging times is a true gift from your heart and helping another in this way can give you purpose and meaning in the world.

However, you can overcare for people which means you spend more time caring for them than you do for yourself. Spending all your thoughts, time and energy on ensuring another is happy, means you may not be spending enough time, love, focus and care on yourself. You may feel more comfortable caring for another, rather than yourself as it can make you feel useful, needed or is simply an unconscious pattern of behaviour.

If you have not been made to feel a priority in the past, it may be hard for you to realise you deserve time, love, care and support. However, there will come a time in your life when you need this and having the courage to ask for and accept it is essential.

Allow yourself to receive the same kindness, love and help that you show to others. Being open to receiving this is essential for your mental well-being; you may feel uncomfortable, possibly undeserving, having this care shown to you, yet learn to accept it.

Sometimes you may reach out to others for help, and they are incapable of giving it to you. Therefore, it is essential to recognise who can give you support and who can't. If you try to get support from people who are unable to give it, due to their own state of mind, then you may become resentful and frustrated.

Being able to ask for help is essential. How comfortable are you in saying the following?

- I am struggling and I need help.
- I don't know where to turn but I need help.
- I don't know what I need now, but I need something.
- Can you listen to me please?

You may not want to bother another person but staying too strong for too long means your mental health can deteriorate as the pressures and burdens build.

Being able to admit you need help is a strength. You will have times in your life when you feel lonely, fed-up or even wondering what the point to your life is. Asking for help is essential and there will always be someone who is ready, willing and able to give it.

SELF-ENQUIRY REFLECTION 8.7

....

Being able to give and receive support ensures a good life balance. Recognise those who suck the energy from you by constantly demanding your time, energy and help. Relationships can be a good balance of giving and receiving love and support.

I have the courage to balance receiving and giving help.

1. On a scale of 0–10 (10 being the maximum) how much positive energy do I give to others?

2. On a scale of 0–10 (10 being the maximum), how much am I able to receive positive energy from others?

3. How much do I overcare for someone and make their happiness my priority?

4. How much do they make my happiness a priority?

5. What support do I need right now, from whom and how can I get this support?

LIFE LESSON

....

Being able to recognise who can give you the right support at the right time is essential. You may struggle to receive this support from a close family or friend, but those in a professional role are often better equipped to help. Sometimes the people who you expect to support you are unable to and recognising this is important for your well-being.

TOPIC 8.8 SAY NO WHEN YOU WANT TO SAY NO

A great way to improve your mental well-being is to have the courage to say no to those demands you don't want to meet. You may not like saying no as the other person may react in a way that makes you feel uncomfortable. Equally, you may feel you are being mean or selfish by saying no to another's requests or demands.

However, being able to say no is called being assertive and is a life-long skill which you can use in your home and work life. Being able to say no to others, often means you are saying yes to yourself which is a form of self-care and improves your mental well-being.

EXAMPLE

Johann accepted his friend's request to attend her house party on Saturday evening. Since then, he has changed his mind but doesn't want to upset Siobhan by now declining the invitation. The night before the party he thinks of every possible reason he can give for not going but his fear of not wanting to upset Siobhan means he attends the party. However, he doesn't enjoy himself and feels resentful that he is spending his evening somewhere he doesn't want to be. He berates himself for being so weak that he cannot say no.

You may have had experiences like the example above, where you said yes at the time and then when you truly thought about it, you wished you hadn't. In this example, Johann had a right to change his mind but fear of not being liked or upsetting his friend made him think he didn't.

You, too, may feel pressure to say yes to requests from your family, friends or partner, as you may be fearful that they will be cross or even sulk with you if you say no. However, knowing you have a right to say no and knowing you can handle their reactions is important for your well-being.

Sometimes others may use emotional manipulation to guilt you into saying yes. Examples of emotional manipulation are:

- you would if you loved me and after all the things I have done for you;
- you are hurting me saying no and I would say yes to you;
- can't you just say yes, this time?
- it is your fault I am upset.

Learning to recognise emotional manipulation can stop you from feeling pressurised to give in and say yes. Owning your *no* means you still say no even when under this pressure and is a sign of being assertive and self-love.

SELF-ENQUIRY REFLECTION 8.8

· ·

Saying no takes courage and once you realise you have a right to say no to others, you will feel less resentful. This is because you are in control of how you spend your time and with whom. The more you learn to do this the happier you will be.

I have the courage to say no.

1. On a scale of 0–10 (10 being the maximum), how comfortable am I saying no to others?

2. Who do I struggle to say no to and why?

3. What do I fear the most about saying no to others?

4. How can I become more comfortable saying no to others?

5. What advice would I give to another on how to say no when they want to say no to another?

LIFE LESSON

· · · · · · · · · · · · · · · · · ·

Being comfortable saying no is a form of self-care. Sometimes you need to say no to yourself, which means stopping behaving in ways which are a form of self-harm, such as unhealthy relationships or putting harmful substances in your body. Have the courage to say no – you deserve to be happy.

TOPIC 8.9 REFRAME SITUATIONS POSITIVELY

When life is challenging, you can find yourself worrying, even obsessing, about a situation. You may reach out to friends or family seeking reassurance that everything is going to work out okay, but often this doesn't make you feel better.

You can obsess about people, outcomes and situations as you want to know how certain events are going to unfold. Often you can have a vision in your mind of how you think you want your life to be and who should be in it. If events are not going according to your plan, you can feel out of control and helpless, leading to unhappiness and upset.

A way you may try to take control is by worrying or obsessing about the situation. This is a form of mental torture as it can make you feel like you are doing something to get the outcome, you want. Yet, as you are aware, no amount of worrying can change an outcome and learning to surrender control, trusting that everything will work out for the best can help you feel much calmer.

It is often only when you look back on an event that you can see why things happened the way they did – why that person stayed away from you, or why you didn't get the job you wanted, for example. What you thought you wanted may not have been the best for you at that time and a bigger plan was in play.

Worrying and overthinking a situation doesn't empower you, so find better ways to take control.

- Reassure yourself that you can and will handle whatever outcome occurs.
- Remind yourself that you have a right to be happy and be treated with respect.
- Tell yourself you are stronger than what you believe yourself to be.
- Repeat 'I let go and trust' and believe the universe has your back.
- Ask yourself, what can I control and what am I not in control of and visualise putting all what you can't control in a rocket and send it to the moon.
- Take positive affirmative action steps to empower you and your future.
- Reflect on what this situation is teaching you about yourself and your life.

Tough situations will happen to you in your life but being able to reduce the amount of time you spend ruminating and worrying will preserve your well-being. Be in the position where you can look back and be proud of the way you handled the situation – in a way which helped you grow and develop as an individual.

SELF-ENQUIRY REFLECTION 8.9

....

I have the courage to stop worrying.

1. On a scale of 0–10 (10 being the maximum), how much do I want to let go of worry, obsessing and ruminating?

2. What are the benefits of worrying, obsessing and ruminating?

3. What would be the benefits of stopping worrying, obsessing and ruminating?

4. What am I worrying about and how can I stop it? (*Do you need to take action to stop you worrying/obsessing about an outcome?*)

5. If I swapped worrying by surrendering or taking action, how would this help me right now?

LIFE LESSON

....

Re-framing situations positively means reflecting on how the universe is trying to empower you. Ask yourself how this situation is helping build inner strength and self-respect. Discern what action you can take to make sure you behave in the most empowering way possible but still allow yourself to feel what you feel.

CHAPTER 9
LIFE AFTER GRADUATION

∙∙

The most empowering choices are made through facing your fears

Rachael Alexander

SCENARIO

∙∙∙∙∙∙∙∙∙∙∙∙∙∙∙∙

Zahra grabbed her homemade sandwich from the work fridge and, keeping her head low, hurried out of the busy chaotic office. Needing to escape the constant phone ringing, she breathed a sigh of relief as the fresh air hit her lungs and she headed off towards the park. Finding a quiet spot, she sat on a bench enjoying the sunshine and solitude and began to unwrap her sandwich, marvelling at how quickly nature could calm her. Within a few minutes, her head stopped pounding and she instantly felt more relaxed.

Hearing her phone ping with a notification, she pulled it out of her bag and smiled at the Facebook memory which had popped up. It was a year since her graduation and there she was, looking ecstatic in her cap and gown, celebrating her degree with university friends. She laughed to herself as she thought back to the celebrations and how happy she had felt that the academic side of university life was over.

Zahra had been a committed student and after graduation had secured an internship as a family lawyer in her hometown. She was passionate about standing up for children's rights and it had seemed the logical career choice. However, a year later and she was seriously wondering if she had made the right decision. It was not that she didn't enjoy her job, but the hours were long, the role was demanding, and she often questioned if she was making a difference due to the failings of the justice system.

Even as an intern she had a huge client list and never seemed to be able to give them all the time and attention they needed, feeling as though she was constantly firefighting. She hadn't expected working life to make her feel so drained and tired all the time, barely having any energy when she returned home, other than collapse on the settee, escaping with a couple of glasses of wine and the latest Netflix series.

She didn't even have time to follow her passion which was reading psychology books as she was tired after work and struggled to focus on the words. This was partly why she made it a priority to have a lunch hour, so she could sit in peace and read her book. Remembering the chapter, she had started yesterday, she pulled the book out of her bag and quickly became engrossed in it. The book *Feel the Fear & Do It Anyway*® by Dr Susan Jeffers was making an interesting point around *'don't protect but correct'* highlighting that many people make a decision and stick to that decision, no matter how unhappy they are. The author was advocating facing your fear of reversing a decision no matter if others disapprove.

Zahra thought about her own life now; where she lived, whom she lived with, the job she did and the lifestyle she had. Did it really bring her the happiness she thought it would or was she sticking with her choices because she feared changing her mind and facing the disapproval of others?

Zahra also witnessed how her older colleagues seemed so unhappy with their lives but didn't seem to change the situation which was causing them emotional pain. One colleague who had worked as a solicitor for over ten years constantly talked about how he wished he had gone into the police force after leaving university. Zahra had gently suggested he explore this option now, but he had replied that his wife wouldn't be happy with the drop in salary and so had to reluctantly stay where he was. Zahra didn't feel it was her place to suggest to him that they could sell the two brand new cars he and his wife drove and downsize from the four-bedroom detached house the two of them lived in. Yet it had made her shudder at how trapped he was by the way he was thinking, his chosen lifestyle and the demands of those around him.

Looking at the time on her phone, she reluctantly put her book away and walked back to work, deep in thought about which decisions she was protecting and not correcting. Making a mental note to finish this chapter in the book that evening, she took a deep breath and walked back into the chaos.

....

Remember ... you've got this

Since secondary school, people around you may have asked you what job you wanted to do. The pressure this can place on you is huge and how are you supposed to know what job you want to do for the rest of your life at such a young age? This ideology is an example of a social construct – a belief that you behave in a certain way.

Some people enter a career at a young age and stay in it even if they are unhappy, often because they think they have no other option or because they have a lifestyle which a salary must fund, such as paying a mortgage or rent, the bills associated and even the cost of raising children. However, Zahra is in a fortunate position where she can make different life choices if she wishes. She made the choice to study law at age 16 when she picked her A-levels, not really knowing if law would suit her as a career. Yet she has tried it and it is not really giving her the happiness or satisfaction she thought it would. Being able to take a step back and recognise that her mental health is suffering is part of her taking responsibility for her life.

Older people in your life may expect you to follow similar paths they have walked, yet you have your own path to walk, and this must be respected. Not needing to fit in or seek approval from others will help you to live authentically. You have a right to seek joy and being flexible and adaptable in changing decisions you have made is key to ensuring this happens. Maturing can be hard, not only for you but for others in your life. Allowing you to have independence and make your own life choices can be challenging for other people, yet they must learn to let go.

It can be hard when others are upset with you but if you ensure you are not being manipulative or cruel in any way, you can follow your own path, knowing you have every right to do so.

Adulthood can be full of new experiences, expectations and responsibilities such as house buying and child-rearing, yet maybe you are in no rush to face these things, nor should you be. But if you do want them now, ask yourself what happiness do you think they will bring? Perhaps look around you at those who have made similar choices and consider whether they are as happy as you would expect. Making conscious choices, free from societal constructs and letting go of what you are 'expected to do', is key to experiencing happiness and living an authentic life.

You may be a free-spirited soul who is not wanting to be weighed down by responsibilities, and this is okay. Many older people, if they were honest, would admit they would make different life choices if they had known the consequences of following the traditions set by society. When you start prioritising your health and well-being over what you feel you ought to do, you will find you live life with more freedom, choices and authenticity. It is your life and you have a right to live it as you choose.

TOPIC 9.1 CHOOSING A FULFILLING CAREER

You may have started your university course with a clear end goal regarding the job you wanted and are on track to achieve this. Alternatively, you may have had a vague idea of the industry you wanted to work in, and your course has clarified your job choice in some way. However, you may have picked a course simply because it seemed interesting and are still no clearer on career choices and you shouldn't worry about this.

Three or four years have passed since starting university and a lot has probably changed for you in many areas of your life. You have probably experienced many highs and lows which have shown you how mentally and emotionally strong you really are. However, the time has now come to consider further study or apply for jobs or internships which may feel scary.

These new life choices may mean moving away from the familiar environment of university and it is okay to feel nervous and apprehensive when catapulted into the unknown. You may not like uncertainty as you don't know what is going to happen to you; few like this feeling of being out of control. Reassure yourself that many people feel this way and show yourself compassion. Your nervousness doesn't mean you have an anxiety disorder, it simply means you are human and experiencing fear because you are treading unfamiliar ground. This is called the journey of life, and as you push through these fear barriers, you become more resilient as an individual and able to handle anything which happens to you. This is true confidence which helps you enjoy life and achieve personal and professional success.

You may even decide you don't want to work in the subject area you have studied for the past three years, and this is okay. However, others may say it is unacceptable, stating you have wasted your time or money. However, changing your mind is an act of courage, as is recognising that you do not want to spend the next 40 years in an industry which is not your passion. Part of adulting is making choices which are right for you and being able to handle others' disapproval if they disagree.

During university you may have discovered an alternative subject which interests you, one which makes you feel excited and passionate, a topic which you want to talk about, even research more in your own time. If you have not had this experience yet do not worry as it will happen one day and when it does you will know you have found your true spiritual purpose. If you want to explore the idea of finding your purpose more, then you may like to consult an astrologer. Astrology is an ancient esoteric science which can help you understand what your soul wants to achieve while you are here on planet earth.

LIFE AFTER GRADUATION

SELF-ENQUIRY REFLECTION 9.1

....

You may have an expectation that you should know the job you want to do for the rest of your life. However, many people spend their lives enjoying exploring different career choices. Staying in the same career all your life, simply because you made the choice at a young age, can feel suffocating and joyless, leading to symptoms labelled as depression.

I have the courage to make the right career choice for me.

1. On a scale of 0–10 (10 being the maximum), how much does the subject I have studied give me passion, meaning and purpose?

2. How am I feeling about finding work related to the subject I have studied?

3. What made me choose the course I have studied for the last few years?

4. What aspects of my studies have I particularly enjoyed?

5. What do I feel are my next steps in finding the right adventure or career for me?

LIFE LESSON

....

Giving yourself permission to change your mind is important as you traverse life. Knowing nothing has been a waste of time, energy or money means you will gain experience from everything which happens to you. Having the courage to follow your interests means you make the right choice for your happiness and potential.

TOPIC 9.2 CONSIDERING FURTHER STUDY

You may know for sure that continuing studying after graduation is the right option for you. However, you may still be undecided, and this indecision may be confusing you.

If you are unsure about the type of job you want, continuing in education can give you more time to decide on a future career and expand your knowledge of a subject, however, it may not be the only option to consider. Asking yourself the following questions may help you to clarify if further study is the right path for you.

1. **Am I considering further study simply because I don't know what else to do?**

While this may seem a good idea, think about the financial investment and the return on this investment? Have you got evidence that further study will improve your job opportunities and increase your salary?

2. **Have I got the self-motivation to continue studying?**

After spending three or four years studying, do you have any motivation to start the process again? Are you happy living the frugal student life for another year or so, especially when many of your friends may be earning money?

3. **Am I trying to prolong university life to avoid the adult world?**

You may have had such a good time at university that you don't want it to end. However, if many of your friends are leaving and you will be alone, will it still be as fun? How many parties dressed as a pirate or nun can you really go to?

4. **Have I considered other options?**

You may be undecided regarding the full-time work you want to pursue, but have you thought about going travelling or setting up your own business? Volunteering or working part time may also be options – it is not student law that you must find a full-time job post-graduation.

5. **Have I found my passion in life?**

Is further study going to lead you towards your passion in life? Does the thought of studying further fill you with joy, passion and excitement? If it doesn't then it may not be the right choice now.

Some people choose not to study further as they doubt their own abilities, however, do not let fear stop you from studying further. If you have the passion, then you will achieve the academic goals you set for yourself.

SELF-ENQUIRY REFLECTION 9.2

....

Choosing the right path for you is important and evaluating all your options is key. You may need to chat with professionals who can help you decide, such as your tutor, coach or careers counsellor. Take your time and maybe consider deferring a course and taking a year out to help give you some thinking space.

I have the courage to choose the right option for me.

1. On a scale of 0–10, how excited am I about the thought of further study?

2. If your score is under 6, why am I considering further study?

3. What other options can I consider?

4. Whom can I talk to which may give me some clarity?

5. What is my gut feeling/heart/intuition telling me to do?

LIFE LESSON

....

Making decisions is an important part of life, however, carrying out research before you decide anything is essential. No decision is ever the wrong decision as you will learn many things about yourself, life and others from the choice you make. However, always research your options carefully, use your intuition and follow the path which you feel will bring you the most joy.

TOPIC 9.3 CONSIDERING MOVING BACK HOME

....

Moving back home could potentially be a challenging time, especially if you have become independent while living away. After being autonomous and making decisions in your life, you may be worried about transitioning back into your home life and being under the same roof and authority as others.

However, with clear communication and a willingness to compromise, home dynamics don't have to be disharmonious, meaning family relationships remain positive and respectful. Of course, be mindful that your family may be unaware of how independent you have become and how confident you are in looking after yourself in the last few years. Perhaps you left for university as a naïve, fearful 18-year-old but are now returning home much more mature and confident in handling life.

Clear communication is needed by all parties to manage expectations, so have an honest conversation with your family about how everyone's needs can be met. For example, your family may be unaware your dietary requirements have changed – such as you now only drink almond milk. Coming to a compromise about who will buy and pay for this milk might be something you need to talk about for example.

Understanding that your family's routines and habits will also have changed meaning you are not a priority, can leave you feeling a little discombobulated. Understanding this and not taking it personally means you remain flexible enough to work with the new routines and not be upset by them.

Considering others is essential. Having 3am Face time sessions with your friends may have been great fun at university but if they have continued and are now waking up the rest of the household then some compromise is needed. It may take a short time to transition but setting an intention of ensuring life at home is both fun and harmonious will help you live happily back with your family.

While moving back home may be wonderful as you may now get your meals cooked and cheap rent, it can often be a sad time as you realise the great experiences you had at university are over. This sadness can seem overwhelming at times, however, just like you transitioned into university from home, you can transition slowly into this next chapter of your life. Allow yourself to feel any emotions you experience.

If you struggle to reach harmony back at home, moving out may have to be considered. This is all part of the maturation process and is simply the next part of your adult journey.

SELF-ENQUIRY REFLECTION 9.3

....

I have the courage to bring my best self back home.

1. What am I looking forward to regarding moving back home?

2. What am I not looking forward to about moving back home?

3. What action can I take to ensure moving back home is the best experience for us all?

4. What will I miss and not miss about student life?

5. What honest conversations do I need to have with those at home?

LIFE LESSON

....

Moving back home is a transition for all involved. Setting strong clear boundaries, being willing to communicate honestly and compromise means family dynamics can be harmonious and respectful.

TOPIC 9.4 HANDLING ASSESSMENT CENTRES AND INTERVIEWS

Completing assessment centres and interviews can be part of the journey to a job and adulthood. This is an exciting time where you can showcase all you have learned.

It is understandable to feel apprehensive and nervous about this new experience. When encountering something for the first time you may feel fear as you do not know what to expect. There may be a part of you which thinks you cannot handle the interviews and assessment centres, but of course, this is untrue. Most people in your situation will be fearful and nervous so do not think it is only you.

Look around the room when you attend the assessment, and you are likely to see anxious faces trying to hide the fear they feel. It is human to feel scared in new situations, but after you have faced your fears by attending the interviews and assessment centre, your fears will dissipate as you realised you could handle it all along. You did not let your fears stop you; in fact, they empowered you, which is exactly the point of fear.

You may fear embarrassment or even failure if you are unsuccessful. However, you are a success, regardless of the outcome, because you faced your fear which is no easy thing to do. Many people allow their fear to win and avoid situations which may trigger their anxiety (fear) but by committing to facing your fears you become more confident.

There is every chance you will be successful and even if you are not, always take the lesson from the experience. After each interview or assessment centre, reflect on how it helped you develop. For example: do you need to prepare more next time? Or speak up more? How did you handle the questioning? Would more preparation on practising responses help you next time? What did you learn about yourself? Do you need to believe in yourself more or shout louder about how good you really are?

Finally, have trust in the universal order of things. You may really want something to happen, such as getting the job, but there may be a bigger picture being played out, that you do not understand. Ask older relatives or friends about something they really wanted to happen which they truly believed was the right thing, but then something else happened which was even better. Trust that the right opportunity will come to you at the right time. The most important thing is to know you can handle anything which comes your way including interviewing news and assessment centres.

SELF- ENQUIRY REFLECTION 9.4

....

Preparation and practice can help ensure you are as successful as you can be. You may have to attend a few interviews before you find the right job for you and of course, the more you attend, the more confident you will become as you realise you can flourish in these situations.

I have the courage to find the best opportunity for me.

1. On a scale of 0–10 (10 being the maximum), how confident am I about attending interviews and assessment centres?

2. What is making me feel anxious – what do I think is going to happen?

3. What advice would I give a wise friend if they told me these fears?

4. What preparation can I do to improve my chances of success?

5. Who can I talk to who can help me feel more confident?

LIFE LESSON

....

Learning to face your fears and push yourself out of your comfort zone is one of the best ways to build confidence. This can seem scary, yet it is more painful to realise that fear stopped you rising to challenges and kept you stuck. You have more chance of achieving your personal and professional goals if you learn to overcome your fears.

TOPIC 9.5 STRUGGLING TO FIND WORK AND CAREER BREAKS

A pressure for students after graduation is finding work in their chosen career. You may be applying this pressure to yourself, or others may be asking you if you have found a job yet. To stop this affecting you, allow yourself to be okay not finding work immediately. Perhaps you started university straight from school and taking some time out for reflection is just what you need right now.

You may want to go travelling after graduation, work part time, volunteer or simply gain experience in a subject which is different from what you studied, and this is okay. What is important is that you are happy in your life. You have probably got another 45 years to work so there really is no rush. People around you may not agree with this and of course may be asking you to contribute to household bills. If this is the case, then some form of work will be needed.

Part of maturing is following your intuition on what feels right for you. You may feel more passionate about volunteering for a charity and working part time which gives you purpose and meaning than landing a full-time job with high pressure and demands. You may even want to change your mind about your future career. For example, you may have studied to be a vet for five years but now decide you want to be a homoeopath. Reversing a decision is an act of courage.

You may be upset if you are unable to find a job you love or feel shame about being unemployed. However, don't get confused between being unemployed and being unemployable. You are not the latter; you are simply waiting to find work which is right for you. There is no failure in saying, this job is not right for me, so I am not going to take it. Of course, if you have financial burdens, then taking some sort of work in the short term is essential. Yet it doesn't mean you will stay there forever.

Take the time to find out about yourself and the type of role you want, and the difference you want to make in the world. You may get more pleasure and joy from helping at the homeless shelter which is far more important than working in a job which is socially approved of.

SELF-ENQUIRY REFLECTION 9.5

....

Being unemployed is not usually the real problem for people, it is the stigma attached to it. However, finding employment straight after university is a social construct that you don't have to follow. Make decisions which are right for you and do not get despondent if it takes time. You are good enough regardless.

I have the courage to find the right employment for me.

1. On a scale of 0–10 (10 being the maximum), how concerned am I about finding employment?

2. What are my real fears about not finding work?

3. How could I talk positively to myself if I am struggling to find the right work?

4. How could I manage others' expectations about this?

5. What else could I do if I do not manage to find work which is right for me?

LIFE LESSON

....

Your life may sometimes not meet your expectations, however, being able to stay resilient and flexible is important for your mental health. Trust what is meant for you will not pass by you and your path will unfold for your highest good. Believe there is a divine cosmic plan at play – having your astrological chart read by a professional astrologer can help you learn more about the cosmic plan.

TOPIC 9.6 AVOIDING THE DEBT TRAP

Student loans are repaid at a low interest rate once you earn over a certain amount. This hopefully does not cause too much concern but being aware of further debt and the impact it can have on your mental health is important.

Some say society encourages you to get into debt through easy credit, so knowing how to avoid this is important. Being in debt means you must make repayments which can create pressure as you must work, and it can also limit your choices in life. For example, in the future, you may want to stop working for some reason such as to have a child, go travelling or even re-train in a different profession, yet you will be unable to do this if you have to make loan repayments. If you fail to make loan repayments, it can affect your credit score in the future.

It is easy to be manipulated by advertisements that encourage you to think you need the latest mobile phone, a better car or even feel pressured to get on the housing ladder. With any of these you are entering a commitment, and even though you think you want that commitment now you may change your mind in the future but will be unable to. It is a good idea to have savings as this then allows you to make different life choices about how you want to live as you are not controlled by debt and repayment plans.

Some people are addicted to buying things as they think it makes them feel good, but this is often a temporary feeling. Many purchases can be emotional – you feel down and buy things to make you feel better. Before you buy anything, get into the habit of asking yourself:

- is this an impulsive purchase to try and make me feel better?
- are there any specific feelings and thoughts am I trying to avoid?
- how is this item a good investment for my future – is it making me a better person?
- do I want this item enough to save up for it or am I willing to go into debt for it?

Having self-discipline and being able to delay gratification are great attributes. Having money saved ensures you don't need to worry about being able to make repayments on past purchases. Being financially independent is a great goal to have – knowing you have enough money to do what you want, when you want, is so empowering and liberating.

Think carefully about any debt you take on – yes you may want a holiday now, but will you really enjoy it if you know you will have to repay it for the next 12 months, long after the tan has faded? Sometimes going into debt is a calculated risk, such as going to university or buying a computer to set up your own business so think carefully about the return on your investment before you make bigger purchases.

SELF-ENQUIRY REFLECTION 9.6

....

Making sound financial decisions is important. Decisions you make now could affect you for the rest of your life. Read up on this subject so you understand more about becoming financially independent as a shortage of money can make life a lot less fun and negatively affect your mental health.

I have the courage to be financially savvy.

1. How much do I spend without really thinking of the long-term financial implications?

2. How much debt am I in and how do I feel about this?

3. What have I been taught about debt from my parents and society in general?

4. How can I start to repay my debt or avoid getting into debt and why would I want to do this?

5. How can I become more financially savvy?

LIFE LESSON

....

Being in debt means you are not free to make choices about how you live your life because you are committed to repaying money. Being able to live debt-free offers peace of mind and gives you more flexibility and freedom, allowing you to make life-affirming choices.

TOPIC 9.7 WORKING 9AM–5PM

. . . .

Since Henry Ford set up his motor factory over 120 years ago, the nine to five working pattern has been the norm. However, being expected to sit in an office, or work from home for eight hours a day may not suit you. You may prefer to sleep in the day, work evenings, split shifts, or even have time off in the week and work weekends. You may even find your true soul calling and work seven days a week as you love your job so much.

Some people like working weekdays nine to five as they have their weekends free; however, this can create Monday morning blues – you feel euphoria on a Friday anticipating not being at work for two days followed by dismay at having a full week of work ahead of you. To live your whole working life with this mentality does not lead to good mental health or an enjoyable life. However because this is the norm for many people, it is easy to think this is the only way to live your life, yet of course it isn't.

In addition, some people are only paid for the hours of nine to five but work many more for no extra pay or reward, which can be demotivating. You may have chosen a career which your family approves of or is the same as one of your parents, thinking it is a safe and secure choice. Yet if your job does not make you feel happy, motivated, and enthusiastic, knowing you are making a difference then you can soon feel stuck in a rut and resentful.

It is therefore important to choose work which inspires and motivates you. This means you work because you love it, rather than being paid to do so.

You may be an innovative entrepreneur who wants to follow your own path in life, working for yourself or teaming up with other friends to set up your own company. While it can be great to get experience in workplaces and learn from others, you may not need this. Having the courage, tenacity and resilience to follow your own ideas can bring you great success and fulfilment.

It is easy to get hooked by a salary rather than job satisfaction. After having little money as a student for the last few years, receiving a pay check at the end of each month can feel great as you are able to buy things when you want to. Enjoy this feeling; however, take lessons from some older people who are in a position where they have to work every month simply to fund a lifestyle and when they take a step back and reflect, they realise the lifestyle is not making them happy, in fact it can make them quite miserable. Yet sometimes they are unable to change their path as they are beholden to monthly debts or are not financially independent. As you traverse your career, encourage yourself to reflect if you are happy with your work, but more importantly ask yourself what can I change if you are not happy. Try to avoid becoming a slave to your salary. Finding work where you make a positive difference to others can give you awesome feelings of satisfaction and fulfillment. In addition, finding work which gives residual income is also a great way to live – this is an income that continues to provide income long after the work is done. You may like to research this idea more.

SELF-ENQUIRY REFLECTION 9.7

....

It is important to listen to yourself. If working nine to five for someone else does not feel right, have the courage to admit this. Making choices which are right for you, regardless of who they may upset, is part of being a mature and healthy adult.

I have the courage to find the right working hours for me.

1. How do I feel about working Monday–Friday 9am–5pm?

2. What would be my preferred hours of working?

3. What work would inspire me and motivate me enough so that it doesn't feel like work?

4. If I don't know what work I would like to do, what am I passionate about or what are my interests?

5. How could I become my own boss and make a business out of something I love doing?

LIFE LESSON

....

It is easy to witness the behaviour of others in society and think you must act in the same way, such as working nine to five. However, you may want to be different and even though this can be a lonely path to explore it frees you to become the person you want to be. Believe that you can live the life you dream of and start to take steps to achieve it.

TOPIC 9.8 UNDERSTANDING SOCIAL CONSTRUCTS

A society often has a set of expectations which people tend to follow as the 'right way to live'. These guidelines may be called traditions, social constructs or social norms, yet they are simply group expectations on how you should live and behave as an individual.

Any deviance from the 'expected way' to live can make you feel different, meaning you wonder if you are wrong or abnormal in some way. For example, people who like to be single can be judged with pity, simply because the expectation by many is that one should be in a relationship. Yet in truth, being single can be empowering as you learn to live independently.

Examples of other social constructs are:

- marriage/divorce/extra-marital affairs;
- having children/not having children;
- working all your life until retirement age/not working;
- following a religion/tradition associated with the religion, eg, christening;
- having a mortgage/renting;
- drinking alcohol/not drinking alcohol.

It is easy to follow social constructs without thinking too much about them. Maybe your family have followed these paths in life, so you think they are the *right* or only ways to live. It is only when someone shows you there are alternate ways to live that you become aware you do not have to repeat others' choices.

None of these constructs is wrong if you want to follow them, the problem occurs when you follow a construct out of fear or because you didn't realise there are different ways to live your life. You may follow the expected way of living as you want to avoid disapproval, not being liked, accepted, rejected or abandoned by another.

Being authentic is knowing you have a right to make choices which will bring you joy. You have a right to be happy and live life on your terms, yet sadly, others in your life may be uncomfortable with your decision to follow your own path. They may fear you will be unhappy with your choices, or they may think they have failed to raise you in the 'right way' simply because you are making different choices to them. However unconditional love means loving you regardless of the decisions you make and if you are unable to receive this from another, then show it to yourself by honouring and owning your decisions. In time, you will find your tribe – those who support you for the way you are choosing to live your life.

SELF-ENQUIRY REFLECTION 9.8

....

I have the courage to explore why I think the way I do.

1. What social constructs have I been raised with, such as traditions I am expected to follow?

2. Which constructs or traditions make me feel unhappy and not want to follow them?

3. How do I think others in my life may feel about this?

4. How will I handle others' opinions on what constructs I want to follow?

5. Who can support me in following my own path?

LIFE LESSON

....

Your mental health can be negatively affected by following social constructs. If you make life choices based on what you think others want, rather than what you want, it can lead to symptoms which have been labelled as depression and anxiety. Have the courage to follow your own path, even if this may appear a lonely path to walk. In time you will see how much confidence and courage this took.

TOPIC 9.9 SERENITY AS A GOAL

You will be encouraged to become a success in many areas of your life, but one area of success which is rarely given focus is experiencing serenity – the state of being calm, peaceful and untroubled. Some refer to it as having inner-peace. This means no matter what happens to you in your life, you deal with it, not allowing anything to steal your personal power as you know you can handle experiencing any feelings evoked by the event. It doesn't mean you don't show any emotion; it means you are comfortable showing whatever emotion is appropriate, but know these emotions are transient and will pass.

Serenity means you:

- do not excessively obsess or worry about events in your life;
- trust in your ability to handle whatever happens to you;
- do not get dragged into dramas or become over emotional about events which are out of your control;
- endeavour to be a positive force in the world;
- trust that a higher power is guiding and protecting you.

The biggest obstacle to experiencing serenity is being fearful and this is why learning to overcome your fears. Once you realise you can handle your fear, you are free from emotional turmoil as you realise how mentally and emotionally strong you are. Displaying an inner strength means you are not afraid of handling any life event; therefore, you are free from worry and live in the state of being calm, peaceful and untroubled – serenity.

Worrying is fear in action and to stop worrying, it is important to write down what your fears are and then list how you can take responsibility to stop these fears affecting your life. Taking action, making a decision or even having the courage to accept what you cannot change are all ways to stop fear affecting your life.

If people around you are not in this same serene state, it can affect your happiness. Your responsibility lies in knowing when to let go of people who don't value this way of living or support and respect the outcomes you want. Whatever decisions you are faced with in your life, always ask yourself if it is likely to bring you serenity. The more decisions you can make from this place, the more likely you will experience a life of contentment, inspiration and joy.

SELF-ENQUIRY REFLECTION 9.9

....

I have the courage to choose serenity as a goal.

1. When have I ever been encouraged to experience inner peace/serenity as a goal?

2. What does the term inner peace/serenity mean to me?

3. What would life be like if I experienced inner peace/serenity?

4. How have I acted in the past which failed to bring me inner peace/serenity?

5. What decisions can I make now which will bring me inner peace/serenity?

LIFE LESSON

....

Experiencing inner peace is rarely given much attention in life and being able to keep it as a focus will aid your mental health. With every decision you make, asking yourself how will this decision bring inner peace means you are much more likely to experience it.

TOPIC 9.10 CREATING A POSITIVE ENVIRONMENT

Creating a positive environment is essential for good mental health. Below are some guidelines to aid your mental health by ensuring your environment is as positive as it can be.

Relationships

Be in relationships which respect and honour who you are. Due to feelings of loneliness, it is easy to attract toxic relationships which can create poor mental health. Have the courage to say no to these types of relationships because you deserve to be loved and treated with respect.

Work

Find work that inspires you where you know you are making a difference. If you are unable to do this currently, ensure your current work environment is fun and you spend time with colleagues and customers who do not drain you.

Embrace your own company

Be comfortable being on your own. If you cannot be in your own company, how do you expect others to love your company? If you do not like to be on your own, reflect on why and overcome your fear of making this happen.

Exercise and fresh air

Find a way of exercising which suits you and if you can do it outside, all the better.

Say no

Be comfortable saying no to things, people and places that steal your joy.

Face your fears

If you do not face your fears, you stay scared. Once you push through these fears you realise you can handle what you think you can't, and the fear disappears.

Avoid negativity

Surround yourself with as much positivity as possible – avoid negative news, people, events, media outlets as much as you can, in fact, anything which doesn't make you feel good.

Rest up

Know when to take a break from work, people or even just the world. Don't think you have to be busy all the time and that rest is for the weak.

Know you have a right to be happy, you are lovable, safe and are of value

Knowing you are unique, lovable and make a difference in the world means you will make choices in the world which bring you joy and happiness.

Healthy choices

Fuel your body with the right contents. Alcohol, drugs and sugary food all negatively affect your mental health.

There are many more ways you can take responsibility to create positive mental health and you will find a list of helpful resources at the back of this book.

SELF-ENQUIRY REFLECTION 9.10

....

Your mental health can start to deteriorate due to the environment you are living in. If you were raised in a traumatic environment, you may not know what a loving, calm environment looks and feels like. This can be healed to ensure you create a positive environment now and will therefore experience good mental health. Releasing hurtful feelings from your past is the healing path of the soul.

I have the courage to take responsibility for my mental health.

1. On a scale of 0–10 (10 being the maximum), how positive is my current environment?

2. How may my environment be affecting my mental health?

3. What can I do to stop this from happening?

4. If I was raised in a traumatic environment, who can I reach out for support to help me heal? (*see resource section*)

LIFE LESSON

....

Your mental health can be affected by your environment, and this is nothing to be ashamed of. What is important is knowing you can take responsibility to improve it, often without the need for medication. Be confident enough to seek support or take action to change your environment in some way.

TOPIC 9.11 BEWARE OF OVERWORKING

....

When you enter a workplace, you can soon become entrenched in the culture of the organisation and overworking may be the norm. People often work more hours than they are paid for and while this can be from a place of motivation, it can also be from a place of fear, duty and obligation.

Overworking can severely affect your mental health. Not achieving a balance of work, rest and play can contribute to feeling stress and pressure, and can impact on your personal life, including relationships.

Prioritising your well-being with strong boundaries and excellent communication skills will help you avoid overworking. When you have healthy self-respect, you will not feel pressurised to behave in the same ways as others. Therefore, if you see overworking is the norm in your organisation, and you do not want to do it, then having an honest conversation with your boss about how you feel is essential. Your mental health is your responsibility.

If you commit 100 per cent effort and energy when you are at work, this means you should commit 100 per cent to the other areas of your life when you leave work. Taking work home with you or answering emails in the evening can interfere with your personal life. Consider why are you doing this. Is it because you love your work or because you fear falling behind or worry what other people will say? If the latter, then you may be susceptible to stress and pressure which, as you fear being judged, won't help your mental health.

More may be expected of you than what you are prepared to give or can give in your job. Being assertive is a skill which means you can speak truthfully, calmly and respectfully to whoever is in charge. Others might also be unhappy with the hours they are working, and you may be the one to lead the change. Perhaps the company is unaware people are overworking and need to recruit more employees? Speaking up is an act of courage.

Working in a career which you love is achievable. As you travel through your career path you can outgrow your job, losing your motivation and you will know when it is time to leave. Staying in one job for all of your life can suit some people, but it doesn't have to suit you. As your soul evolves, it will want more challenge and stimulation, and leaving one situation to start another may give you the excitement you are craving. It takes courage to walk your own path, but it is a soul-enhancing experience.

SELF-ENQUIRY REFLECTION 9.11

· ·

Working too many hours is an easy trap to fall into, especially when you are new to a job or company. It may be the norm but consider carefully if you really want to overwork and be aware that your mental health may start to suffer.

I have the courage to not overwork.

1. On a scale of 0–10 (10 being the maximum), how comfortable am I saying no to working more hours than the company originally stated?

2. What would stop me from saying no?

3. On a scale of 0–10 (10 being the maximum), how much do I prioritise my mental health and well-being over the hours I work?

4. How would overworking affect my mental health?

5. How could I explain to my superiors that I value my mental health and overworking is not contributing to it?

LIFE LESSON

· · · · · · · · · · · · · · · · · · · ·

Balancing the time and energy you give to all areas of your life contributes to great mental health. If you focus a large proportion of your time on work only, you miss out on creating memories with loved ones, experiencing joyful feelings and fully embracing all life has to offer.

TOPIC 9.12 EMBRACING LIFE AT THE RIGHT PACE FOR YOU

Now you are leaving university, you may feel pressurised to enter the next stage of adulthood, such as working full time, earning a good salary, finding a committed relationship and even purchasing a house or moving out of home. Of course, if you want to do all these things consciously and willingly then embrace the adventures.

However, you may not want to follow this expected route and following your own path is part of being an independent, autonomous adult. You may have different dreams and goals from others so have the courage to follow your own path.

There can be a lot of pressure from others to live life the way they expect you to live and to the timeframes they set. But you do not have to do this and now is a good time to know you can make different choices to others.

Getting a mortgage and having children means your life irreversibly changes, even if you think it won't. Society can often judge people who do not want to follow the conventional way of living, but you may be a free-spirited soul and don't want these responsibilities and that is okay. You may want to explore the world at your pace and not at the pace others dictate. You may wait until you are in your fifties to settle down or have no desire to own a house or have children, and this is okay. To walk into responsibilities before you are ready for them may make you feel stuck, trapped and unhappy. Therefore, giving yourself permission to follow your own heart is key.

It is also easy to compare yourself with others, such as your university friends and believe you must follow the same route as them at the same pace. Of course, this is untrue and trust that your path is the right path to walk at the pace you want to walk it.

There is a saying: whatever the majority is doing, do the opposite. Sadly, some people have been conditioned to live their life in a certain way, yet when you look closer, you can see these people are unhappy with the life they live and feel trapped, thinking they cannot reverse decisions they once made. This is often because many have been raised to value the materialistic side of life and have never been taught to listen to their soul or allow their spirit to lead them. However, you have the chance to do this, before you become trapped into living a certain way. The film *The Matrix* with Keanu Reeves and Carrie-Anne Moss is a good example of living your life on your terms and living free from the matrix.

SELF-ENQUIRY REFLECTION 9.12

....

Having the courage to walk your path at your own pace is important and will help you make the right life choices for you. Give yourself time to think about what you want, rather than giving in to pressure from others, including society. You have a right to make choices which make you happy.

I have the courage to walk my own path at my own pace.

1. On a scale of 0–10 (10 being the maximum), how much do I feel pressurised to live my life in a certain way?

2. On a scale of 0–10 (10 being the maximum), how much do I feel overwhelmed about starting to live life as a grown-up?

3. If could do anything right now, what would I like to do?

4. How pressurised do I feel to do something that I don't really want to do?

5. Who can I speak to who may be able to help me? (*life coach, counsellor, parent, family friend, role-model*)

LIFE LESSON

....

There may be someone in your life who is telling you how to live your life. However, you do not have to follow others advice, and this is simply their opinion. Making your own judgements and owning the consequences of your decisions is part of maturing and becoming an adult.

TOPIC 9.13 LETTING GO OF STUDENT LIFE

The last three or four years you spent at university will be a part of your life that you will probably never forget. You may have achieved a great deal academically and personally; probably made some great friends and become clearer about the type of person you want to be and the difference you want to make in the world.

After the graduation celebrations have ended and you have said goodbye to your friends, you may feel a little lost, sad and alone. If you have returned home and re-connected with old school or college friends who have not had the university experience, you may feel distant and disconnected from them.

Leaving university can be a time of grief as you mourn the loss of routines, friends, habits, relationships, interests, even your own living accommodation. Moving from studying x number of hours a week to working a 40-hour week can be a shock to the system. And while the salary can be comforting, having reduced freedom and flexibility can feel strange at the beginning. When something finishes which has brought you pleasure it is understandable to feel bereft, and your body may release these feelings by wanting to cry and be alone.

Just as going to university was a huge transition, leaving is another one. Therefore, show yourself compassion and nurture yourself. You have worked hard to be in this position and now is the time to congratulate yourself on the degree you have achieved while still acknowledging these feelings of loss.

Being a responsible adult means honouring your feelings and making choices which are right for you.

Like Zahara in our scenario at the start of this chapter, you may be realising that you do not feel fulfilled in the career you have chosen. This is understandable, and it takes courage to admit you may be ready for a change. You were probably 16 when you made your career choice, picking A-levels to help you enter university. You are a different person now and will probably have changed in many ways, which of course is the point of life. Your soul will direct you in life by giving you nudges through your feelings – this is your guidance system and needs to be listened to. The only thing which can stop you following this internal guidance is fear, fear of being judged, disapproved of, criticised and even ridiculed. However you develop self-confidence and self-belief by overcoming this fear and making decision which you know in your heart are right for you. Other people will always judge you, yet knowing you had the strength and courage to make life choices which are right for you is an authentic way to live.

SELF-ENQUIRY REFLECTION 9.13

∙∙

If you need to, allow yourself the time to process the loss of university life. You may feel strange in your new job, however, it may simply be a case of fearing the unknown which is making you feel uncomfortable. Give yourself a period of time to adjust but if you still think your job is not right for you, then look to make changes.

I have a right to let go of student life at my pace.

1. On a scale of 0–10 (10 being the maximum), how sad do I feel that my university experience is over?

2. What are my happiest memories while at university?

3. What have I learned about myself while at university?

4. Now I have left university, what will I miss the most?

5. What do I need from myself and others to help me transition into the next stage of my life?

LIFE LESSON

∙∙∙∙∙∙∙∙∙∙∙∙∙∙∙∙∙∙∙∙∙

Your life is like a book and the different life events you will encounter are akin to its chapters. University was one chapter in your book, and hopefully, you will have learned many things about yourself and others. Take the lessons and move on, ready to live your next exciting chapter.

CHAPTER 10
AN INTRODUCTION TO CHAPTER 10

....

HOPE
Hold On, Pain Ends

Author unknown

This final chapter of the book deals with the confusing subject of mental health. However, to help remove some of this confusion, topics are discussed to help you understand your mental health better.

I understand my mental health as the way I think, feel and behave, which can fluctuate daily. Sometimes I think and feel great which leads me to behave in inspiring and empowering ways. However, there have been times in my life when the opposite was true; harmful thoughts and an unhelpful belief system led to feelings of despair and despondency, resulting in me behaving in ways harmful to myself. Sometimes I would think what's the point in me being here and would even think my son would be better off if I wasn't alive anymore. Thankfully at these times, because of my training, I knew to reach out and find someone who would give me a little bit of hope to believe there was a reason to stay. I later learned these are known as dark nights of the soul; they are painful but they do pass. You too will have these at times, and learning more about them will help you on your spiritual journey.

There are many ways to help a person who is suffering with these dark times, when they are suffering with their mental health, and as a spiritual psychologist, the ideas I suggest for healing in this chapter may be different from what you have heard before. I offer an alternative view to the mainstream narrative, and I hope that for some of you these ideas will resonate as the truth.

However sometimes, like me, you might feel so low that you don't have the energy to implement any of the suggestions in this book and all you need at that moment is someone to listen to you, to give you hope, a reason to get through the day or night. If you are feeling this way right now, then please reach out to someone, just like I have done in the past.

UNDERSTANDING MENTAL HEALTH

There are many great organisations such as Samaritans and Nightline which are staffed by caring individuals who want to help you. There are also medical professionals, and your university can also offer support via online guides, your tutor, student services and pastoral support so please reach out to someone who is waiting to help you. One thing I know for sure is that tough times do pass; it just doesn't feel that way at the time. This is one moment in time, you can handle it and you will come out the other side of this dark tunnel you are in.

One of the biggest challenges many humans face is being overwhelmed by their emotions, especially the darker ones, and understandably you become scared of feeling this way. Yet your power lies in being able to handle all your emotions, and the more you can learn to transcend your pain by knowing you can handle feeling this way, the more resilient you become. I know this because a few years ago I suffered heartbreak like I had never suffered before and at times believed the emotional pain would never end, and yet with continued self-development work, energetic healing and some supportive people around, I healed. The experience was such a soul gift (even though it didn't feel like it at the time) because I now know that I can handle such deep pain again. The pain passed because i understood what the pain was trying to teach me about myself and I learned the soul lesson. I survived it just like I know you can as long as you have the right tools around you. Of course, if the emotional pain is making you think you do want to be alive anymore, then reach out, just like I have done at times, being mindful of what intuitively feels the right intervention for you. Sources of support which have helped me over the years are listed at the end of the book.

You are important, you do matter, and you need to be here, so please reach out for help and support.

UNDERSTANDING MENTAL HEALTH

···

Take care of your body, it's the only place you have to live.

Jim Rohn

SCENARIO

··············

Suddenly jolting awake from his comatose state, Jay groaned as he slowly opened one eye, painfully becoming aware of his dry mouth, pounding head and an overwhelming sense of nausea. Becoming more conscious by the second, he raised his aching head from the pillow and wondered where he was and, more importantly, who the hell the blonde-haired girl was next to him.

Feeling grateful as he spotted his phone on the bedside table, he looked at the time and groaned again as he realised he was late for a meeting with his tutor. Briefly wondering if he should skip it, but then remembering he had missed the last one, he quietly extracted himself out of the bed trying not to wake the mystery girl beside him. Experiencing a flashback from the night before, he vaguely recalled meeting her at a house party but for the life of him couldn't remember her name. Feeling slightly ashamed he crept out of the door, carrying his trainers in his shaking hands.

He plucked up the courage to look at his phone to see how many missed calls he had from his girlfriend. '*Shit*', he muttered as he realised it was 26, wondering how he was going to explain this one. He knew she would be panicking big time and felt a growing sense of desperation realising her anxiety might have caused her to self-harm.

If truth be told, Jay felt a burden of responsibility as he continually tried to be the mentally strong one in their relationship and support her mental health. But he also knew the odd drunken one-night stand eased this pressure but it was only a temporary respite. In fact, the pressure Jay was feeling recently about everything in his life was making him party harder and even use more weed and, worryingly, the anti-depressants his doctor had issued last year didn't seem to be helping as well as they once had.

He hadn't been sure about taking the medication but the doctor advised that Jay was probably depressed after the death of his father a few months earlier and so it seemed the right thing to do, especially when the doctor indicated it would help Jay focus on his studies. And the pills had seemed to work for a few months, as the uncomfortable feelings he felt had eased his life had become more manageable again. Granted he sometimes felt a bit spaced out, but having a drink and the university party lifestyle allowed him to cope.

The constant heartache Jay felt after losing his dad five months ago and seeing the anguish in his mum's face, along with hearing his little sister cry out in her sleep each night, had made Jay withdraw into himself, refusing to talk to anybody about how he felt. Not wanting to burden his mum with his feelings, believing she had enough to deal with, no one knew how much Jay was struggling to cope. Occasionally in his darkest moments, he had thoughts about not being alive anymore but the guilt of how it would affect his family made him not act on his thoughts.

··

Remember ... you've got this

Your mental health is simply the way you think, feel and behave daily. As an adult, your mental health can be affected by many things. Contributory factors include your parent's genetics, brain development while in your mother's womb, the environment you experienced as a child including home and school, how well you processed your emotions when faced with traumatic and painful experiences such as accidents, trauma, bullying or bereavement, and finally, how safe you felt in the environment you were raised in. Of course, your mental health can also be affected by current events and circumstances too.

It is important children and teenagers are taught how to positively deal with challenging life events such as bereavement and bullying in order that they learn emotional intelligence and are able to handle life. Then, when faced with the demands and responsibilities of adult life, they can think, feel and behave in empowering ways, which means their mental health will not suffer.

Understandably trauma, loss and challenging life events can be emotionally painful and can cause you to feel hopeless, which makes reality difficult to deal with. When you feel so low, you may look to relieve these uncomfortable feelings in some way such as with alcohol, drugs or tablets. Of course, alcohol and drugs are not effective coping strategies as they are addictive which can add to any existing problems.

While some psychiatric drugs have been shown to help, they are not always the only available solution. This is because the tablet alone might not help you change the life event which is causing you to feel a certain way or caused you to feel a certain way in the past. Being able to naturally heal what caused you emotional pain in the past and learning how to become more able in dealing with the challenges you are facing today can be an empowering solution.

Many doctors encourage patients to seek additional psychological interventions such as counselling and other talking therapies to help process and release painful emotions or to seek support in dealing with the life event which is causing them to feel a certain way. They discuss with the patient the pros and cons of taking medication, helping the patient make an informed choice whether medication is right for them at this time.

Jay has experienced a bereavement and it would appear he didn't have the most appropriate support to help him grieve when his dad passed. Due to his empathic, sensitive nature, he didn't want to burden other people with his feelings and was more concerned with soothing his loved ones. However, this means he has not allowed himself to fully grieve the death of his father and has failed to release the emotional pain he felt. Talking to a bereavement counsellor at the time of his father's passing could have helped Jay process and understand why he was feeling the way he did.

When someone is empathetic and neglects their own feelings, they often take the role of a caregiver for another, meaning the dynamic of Jay and his girlfriend's relationship is not as healthy as it could be. His girlfriend is also suffering, needing professional help and Jay is not equipped, due to his own emotional pain, to effectively support her. While he can be a listening ear, he is not qualified to help her explore why she is self-harming. Because of the pressure Jay is under, he is using the only coping strategies he knows – numbing his feelings through drinking and also engaging in some self-sabotaging behaviours such as one-night stands.

Jay needs time to heal, and this would be achieved through processing the emotional pain of his father's death – he may be afraid of feeling this pain, thinking he can't handle it, but of course, he can. No wonder Jay thinks about ending his life as it's not only devoid of joy, true connection and happiness but he is feeling lonely, stressed and burdened. However, if Jay can seek the right support he can release his grief, slowly begin to heal and make some healthy choices around his life and current relationship. Making an informed choice about the use of psychiatric tablets is also important so visiting his doctor to talk about this, as well as additional forms of healing such as referral to counselling or a support group, will help him. If you can relate to Jay's scenario, there are books listed in the resource section from authors who have conducted scientific studies surrounding the use of psychiatric tablets and offer alternative suggestions on how to handle the times when your mental health is not as good as it could be. However, there is never one size fits all when it comes to treating mental health, and if you feel medication and some sort of psychological therapy is the right avenue for you to take, then this is your choice. Simply be aware of the possible side-effects and withdrawal procedures.

TOPIC 10.1 WHY DO I STRUGGLE WITH MY MENTAL HEALTH?

'*Mental health*' is a term which describes how you *think*, *feel*, and *behave*. Your mental health can fluctuate depending on what has happened to you in your past and what you are experiencing in the present day. It is not uncommon to sometimes experience symptoms of poor mental health as life can be extremely challenging sometimes.

When you have good mental health, you have positive, affirming thoughts, experience feelings of love, connection and joy meaning you make life-affirming, empowering choices and increase your chances of reaching your soul potential. A way to experience good mental health is learning how to reframe your thinking from negative to positive because negative thoughts lead to unhappy feelings and self-sabotaging behaviour.

> For example, if you *think* a negative thought, such as I am going to fail my exam, you may *feel* hopeless meaning you want to give up and stop revising. Your negative thought has led to a low mood which has resulted in self-sabotaging negative *behaviour*. Yet, by affirming, my best is enough and I pass my exams (positive thought) means you have switched your negative thought to a positive one and this helps you feel more empowered, meaning you will continue with your revision (positive behaviour).

Being able to switch negative thoughts to positive thoughts can greatly improve your mental health; however, it is not always possible, and you should not berate yourself if you are unable to do this. You may need help in finding ways to think more positive and your university will be able to offer you support. In addition, the further reading and resources section offers ideas.

For some people, thinking positively can be hard to do as you may have been pro-grammed to react fearfully, especially if you experienced any of the following:

- neglect or abuse of any kind – sexual, physical, mental or emotional;
- being shouted at and/or given verbal messages such as '*you are stupid*';
- being criticised, controlled and coerced – told who to be and how to behave;
- trauma caused by upsetting experiences such as being raised in an argumenta-tive home, bereavement or bullying;
- not taught to believe or trust in yourself – seeing yourself as flawed in some way;
- a perceived withdrawal of love and nurturing from those who cared for you.

It may be upsetting to learn that your past has caused you to react fearfully, how-ever, this awareness means you can now start to reprogramme your thinking, meaning your mental health can and will improve.

This process of moving from a painful place of mental suffering to having healthy thoughts and experiencing loving feelings is your spiritual birthright.

SELF-ENQUIRY REFLECTION 10.1

Learning how to improve your mental health is the key to enjoying life and some believe true success is living with great mental health, free from worry and stress. These questions share insight into how you can take responsibility to live free from experiencing poor mental health.

I have the courage to investigate my past.

1. On a scale of 0–10 (10 being the maximum), how much do I suffer daily from negative thinking and uncomfortable feelings?

2. Have I self-diagnosed myself as having a mental health disorder and if so, how may this self-diagnosis be disempowering me?

   You may have been given a mental health diagnosis and prescribed psychiatric medication by a doctor. However, medication might not fully address the core issue which caused your symptoms to appear in the first place. It is highly recommended you explore your feelings with a professional surrounding the event which caused you to suffer.

3. How may my childhood/teenage experiences have resulted in me having poor mental health as an adult? (*Have you experienced any negative experiences growing up such as bullying at school, an argumentative home life, abusive relationships?*)

4. What self-development tools can I access to reprogramme my current way of thinking? (*Your university will have online guides available*)

5. Who else can I reach out to for support to help improve my mental health? (*Tutor, lecturer, counsellor, friend, parent, internet, doctor*)

LIFE LESSON

You can start to suffer with poor mental health at any age. This is not weak and it is important you are comfortable in reaching out for help. Support from others can help you become self-aware, reflecting on how your thoughts, feelings and behaviour are contributing to poor mental health.

TOPIC 10.2 MY MENTAL HEALTH HAS FURTHER DECLINED SINCE STARTING UNIVERSITY

Moving to university may mean you have lost the support of your close friends and/or your mental health team which is making you feel more unsettled. It is therefore crucial you reach out for help and find a new support system. You may have arrived at university with an existing mental health diagnosis and the unfamiliar university environment can trigger your symptoms due to you feeling fearful which leads to you experiencing symptoms of anxiety.

Once you have settled into a routine at university and are feeling supported and reassured, it may be a good time to explore what causes you to feel the way you do. If you have been given psychiatric medication in the past to manage your mental health without exploration as to why you started to experience such symptoms, then it may be a good time to do this.

Alternatively, you may have self-diagnosed with a mental health diagnosis such as anxiety and therefore you may self-soothe or self-manage your emotional pain each day through the following:

- relying on non-prescription drugs or excess alcohol consumption;
- self-harming such as cutting yourself or purging with food;
- eating too much of the wrong foods such as those with a high sugar content;
- excessive exercise or other obsessive-compulsive behaviours;
- unhealthy attachments or co-dependent relationships.

While these may seem to help you manage day-to-day life, in the long run, they may be making your mental health and, in some cases your physical health, worse. The key to improving your mental health at university is finding someone who understands what you are experiencing and who can teach you how to change unhelpful coping mechanisms into more helpful thoughts and behaviours.

It is useful if this is a medical professional such as a trained counsellor, but other resources such as psycho-spiritual groups, self-help books, motivational influencers, podcasts, and YouTube videos can also provide inspiration. Even though you may have struggled with your mental health prior to university, this does not mean you have to struggle with it throughout your university experience and beyond. Being able to heal past traumas and learning more positive ways to cope can help you live free from poor mental health. Do remember that if you are on medication and want to withdraw then you must consult your doctor who can ensure you do this safely and can suggest alternative interventions.

While you may still have challenging days you can become emotionally intelligent and learn to handle the ups and downs of life, meaning you live life authentically and empowered free from chemical stimulants.

SELF-ENQUIRY REFLECTION 10.2

....

While a mental health diagnosis can help you understand why you feel the way you do, it can potentially disempower you, preventing you from trying new experiences, enjoying life and achieving your potential.

I have the courage to explore my diagnosis.

1. What diagnosis have I been given in my past, or have I given myself? (*eg I suffer from anxiety, I have OCD, I am depressed*)

2. How, on reflection do I think this diagnosis may be disempowering me? (*eg You may say, I can't do that because of my anxiety or 'it may bring my depression on'*)

3. What self-development work, if any have I conducted in the past to help me understand why I feel the way I do?

4. Who or what could help me conduct some self-enquiry work to help me explore my past?

5. What psycho-spiritual techniques could help me understand how to manage my mental health better? (*see resource section*)

LIFE LESSON

....

If you have experienced an emotionally painful past or are experiencing challenges in your life now, then it is understandable you are struggling. Healing repressed emotions from your past and understanding how to manage your mental health means you can live with love, peace and joy, free from poor mental health.

TOPIC 10.3 I AM CONSIDERING TAKING ANTI-DEPRESSANTS AS I FEEL SO LOW

Sometimes you may feel so low, overwhelmed, hopeless and helpless that you will consider taking psychiatric medication to help you feel better. Your feelings may seem so strong and debilitating that they are stopping you from enjoying life. It is to be commended that you are willing to reach out, ask for help and consider medication as an option.

It is an act of bravery to admit you need help, and for some medication is the only intervention offered. However, some young people may feel medication is not right for their body and want to seek alternative solutions. Of course, some medication can be very helpful, but there are also alternative or additional options you can explore. Often the medication can help make you feel better, but it may not tackle the root cause of why you feel the way you do. What is happening in your life right now to make you feel this way, or what has happened to you in your past to make you feel this way? You didn't leave your mother's womb with the symptoms you feel now, so when did they start? Being a university student can be challenging at times and this is why accessing psychological support is so important as there are people who can help you make sense of why you are thinking, feeling and behaving the way you do.

You may feel low due to adverse events which occurred in your childhood, and these have caused you to suffer emotionally. As a child you may not have had your emotional needs met or been able to express yourself authentically, meaning your feelings have never been expressed and are waiting to be released. With the right help and support, you can learn to release these feelings and not feel so overwhelmed by the pain meaning poor mental health symptoms may disappear as you learn to increase your emotional intelligence.

You may have self-diagnosed yourself with anxiety or depression. While these labels may explain your symptoms, they do not explain why you are experiencing them. There are many people who can help you explore alternative ways to heal such as counsellors, psychotherapists, hypnotherapists, astrologers and energy healers such as reiki and crystal healers. While some people may be sceptical of these healing modalities, it is often the people who have never tried them and you should be mindful of this when listening to other's opinions on the use of these natural healing modalities.

Discuss with your doctor the benefits and side effects of any psychiatric medication you are prescribed along with any risks such as dependency and withdrawal. Make sure you have all the information necessary to help you make an informed decision on the right treatment plan for you including any referrals to outside support. Remember a doctor has been trained in the medical model and is likely to offer this. It is simply a different model from the psycho-spiritual techniques I offer in this book. As an adult, you can decide for yourself which model suits you best: a mixture of both models may even be appropriate. Talking to a range of professionals about the different ways the interventions work will help you make an informed choice.

SELF-ENQUIRY REFLECTION 10.3

....

While you may think medication is the only solution to help you feel better, there are also other options which you can consider, and conducting independent, informed research is a worthwhile exercise. The resources section lists some books by academics which you may find of interest.

I have the courage to seek holistic support.

1. On a scale of 0–10 (10 being the maximum), how much am I considering taking medication to help minimise the way I feel?

2. Do I believe medication is the only option for feeling better?

3. Do I understand the benefits and possible side effects of psychiatric medication?

4. What other solutions are available to help me feel better?
   (*Counsellor, internet, energy practitioners, higher-self, social media, self-help*)

5. How do I feel about exploring other solutions?

Medication and therapy can be prescribed together. If you want to reduce your medication you must take advice from a trained professional such as a doctor or psychiatrist.

LIFE LESSON

....

While medication can help people traverse a challenging life experience, it may not always be the only option. Sometimes taking medication in the short term while exploring a more holistic path can be helpful. What is important is conducting research to find out the right intervention which will help you heal long-term.

TOPIC 10.4 WHY DO I WITHDRAW INTO MYSELF WHEN I FEEL OVERWHELMED?

....

When you feel overwhelmed with life, it is understandable you withdraw into yourself. This means you do not want to see or speak to anyone, wanting to be left alone with no interruptions from the outside world. You may avoid people, places and situations which place pressures and demands as you feel unable to cope. You can think it is easier for yourself and others if you are left alone.

Any noise, interruption or request of any kind can simply feel too much for you to handle. You may feel angry, sad or generally apathetic about life, and your own space feels like the safest option for you.

While there is a time and a place to have your own space to just be, if you withdraw too much it can make you feel worse. This is because, at your core, you need to receive love and be nurtured in some way. To feel alone, unloved and unsupported is a harsh place to be, making you feel helpless and possibly not wanting to be alive anymore.

The biggest act of courage you can take now is to do the opposite, so reach out to another and tell them how you are feeling and what you need, which may be:

- someone to listen to you – a shoulder to cry on;
- encouragement, guidance and hope;
- nurture, love and kindness;
- someone to tell you everything is going to be okay.

Expressing to someone how you feel and what you need at this moment is a vulnerable yet assertive act. If the first person you reach out to is unable to give you what you need, then continue until you find someone who can. This may need to be a someone who is trained in listening and the resource section offers sources of support. You have a right to receive kindness from another to help you. Remember you are here to make a positive difference in the world, it just doesn't feel that way right now.

Tough times do pass, but while you are going through the challenging time it can feel like it will never end as you can see no light at the end of the tunnel. However, believe there is a bigger picture at play to your life, and even though you may not understand why you feel the way you do, trust the universe has your back. Your soul never asks for more than it can handle, and it is often in the most painful times that we discover the strength we have inside. You may like to consult an astrologer to see why you are experiencing tough times and the lessons your soul is wanting to learn. While this may not take the pain away, it does help to know when your feelings are likely to subside.

SELF-ENQUIRY REFLECTION 10.4

....

Simply recognising that you are withdrawing from others is great awareness. Knowing how to stop this and reach out for support is key to your well-being. These questions will help you identify why you withdraw and what to do differently next time you want to do this.

I have the courage to reach out to others.

1. On a scale of 0–10 (10 being the maximum), how much am I withdrawing right now?

2. What is happening in my life to make me want to withdraw?

3. How does withdrawal into myself make me feel?

4. What would reaching out to another give me instead?

5. Whom can I reach out to and what do I need right now from them? (*Tutor, counsellor, lecturer, friend, parent, doctor, internet, higher power, energy healer, external support group?*)

LIFE LESSON

....

Sometimes you can self-sabotage your happiness by withdrawing into yourself rather than reaching out for support, love and kindness. Even reading positive books or listening to positive music or podcasts can help you feel better about yourself and life. This unhappy time will pass – have faith. Asking for help is an act of courage and you are worthy of experiencing kindness and love.

TOPIC 10.5 HOW DO I STOP MY FEELINGS OVERWHELMING ME?

As a human you have the ability to use logical reasoning and experience feelings; both can help you navigate your way successfully through life. Feelings are a fantastic biological intervention because they give meaning to your life – to experience joy, happiness, hope, love and peace makes life worth living. Other feelings such as fear, anger, sadness and apathy are not perceived in such a positive light, however, all feelings are worthy of respect because this is how you are guided through your life.

For example, when someone you love passes away, it is understandable you may feel upset. Therefore, you may cry which is simply your body releasing your emotional pain. Alternatively, if you feel anger, this may indicate a need to protect yourself. Every feeling is an intuitive messenger and discerning how they are guiding you is important for your future success and happiness.

You may not have been taught to listen to these intuitive emotional messages (feelings) and this may mean you are unable to access important guidance such as 'stop doing that' or 'this person is not good for you to be around' meaning you may be making unhealthy life choices.

In the past, you may have felt so overwhelmed by your thoughts and feelings that you may have taken psychiatric medication, which is understandable. However, the more you access psychological support to help you understand your thoughts and feelings, the more you will learn to handle challenging situations, reducing the need for medication.

It is also important not to label your feelings as positive or negative as you may not allow yourself to feel what you perceive to be a *negative* feeling such as anger or sadness. All feelings have a right to be felt and serve a purpose. When you feel a certain way, learn to ask yourself:

'What am I *thinking right now* to experience these feelings?'

If you are having negative thoughts about yourself and the world, then you will experience negative feelings and replacing these with more positive thoughts allows you to balance your emotions, preventing you from becoming overwhelmed. Your university may offer online guides to help you do this, and you can find further resources at the back of the book to help you explore this empowering subject in more detail. Energy healing can help release a build of emotions which may be sending your energy system out of balance. It is worth exploring these modalities to help you re-balance.

SELF-ENQUIRY REFLECTION 10.5

....

To learn how to balance your logic and feelings is a skill which needs practice. Sometimes you can become overly emotional which halts your logical self from working. Equally you may not listen to your feelings meaning you miss the intuitive messages that are needed for your well-being.

I have the courage to experience all my feelings.

1. On a scale of 0–10 (10 being the maximum), how much do my feelings overwhelm me?

2. How does it feel when I get overwhelmed by my feelings?

When you feel overwhelmed by your feelings, you're thinking has probably slipped into the negative. See if you can identify the negative thoughts which are causing your negative feelings.

3. How, if at all have, I been taught to see my feelings as guidance?

4. Give an example of how a recent negative thought has led to a negative feeling then reframe this negative thought into a positive thought and see how you then feel.
   (eg Negative thought = I have no friends = feel lonely
   Positive thought = I have a dear friend from school = feel comforted)

5. Where can I learn more about how to reframe my negative thoughts
   (Books, podcasts, counsellors, doctor, YouTube, websites, forums, groups)

LIFE LESSON

....

Learning to balance your logic and feelings can help you make important decisions which will make life more meaningful. Not fearing your feelings is an important lesson. Becoming more self-aware about how your thoughts are linked to your feelings is a great personal skill to have, and organisations also welcome emotional intelligence.

TOPIC 10.6 WHY AM I STRUGGLING TO SLEEP?

Many people, at some point in their life will struggle with their sleep routine. You may have trouble falling asleep in the evening, disrupted sleep throughout the night or waking very early. Sometimes this may be due to the life choices you are making which may not be beneficial for your sleep pattern, such as excess alcohol intake or working late into the evening, yet at other times it may simply be the demands of life or even your body adjusting to the natural rhythms and moon cycles of our planet.

To give yourself the best chance of sleeping well it is useful to investigate what may be disrupting your sleep and how you can improve it.

Stop worrying about things you cannot control

Worrying about life events can stop you sleeping because *worry* is fearful thoughts which cause adrenaline and cortisol hormones to be released into your body. These hormones flood you with energy and stop you from sleeping. The way to stop these hormones from keeping you awake is to write down what you are worrying about and ask yourself, 'What action can I take to stop myself worrying about this?', then make a list of what you can do to resolve the situation. If you are unable to think of any solutions, then acknowledge this and imagine surrendering your worry to the divine intelligence to resolve.

Have a '*fuck it*' bucket

Often, the issue you are worrying about is not worth your time and effort. Ask yourself, '*Will I be worrying about this problem in six months' time?*' If the answer is no, then slam dunk your worry into a real or imaginary fuck it bucket!

Remove toxicity from your body

Toxic products such as caffeine, sugar, alcohol and non-prescription drugs can prevent you from sleeping. Even though alcohol can act as a sedative and make you sleepy, it prevents you from experiencing important sleep patterns. Making empowered choices regarding what you put in your body is an act of self-love and sleep is one of the most important activities for your well-being and mental health.

Meditation

Using meditation and visualisation apps can help you fall asleep and get quality sleep for longer (see the further reading and resources section).

Medication

You may think about visiting your GP to be prescribed some sleeping tablets; however, remember these might not treat the root cause of why you are struggling to sleep and can have side effects. Talking to your doctor about what may be causing you to not sleep may be useful as they may be able to refer you to a sleep clinic or meditation group for example.

SELF-ENQUIRY REFLECTION 10.6

....

Being unable to sleep can severely affect your mental and emotional well-being and developing a healthy sleep pattern can improve the chances of academic success. These questions will help you identify how you can make healthier choices to improve your sleep.

I have the courage to find suitable ways to relax and fall asleep.

1. On a scale of 0–10 (10 being the maximum), how poor is my sleeping now?

2. What do I think is causing me to not sleep properly?

3. If I am not sleeping due to worry, what action can I take to stop the worrying?

4. What empowering choices (which you may not have tried before) can I try to help me sleep properly?

5. What or who else could help improve my sleep pattern?
   (*Online resources, professional, tutor, lecturer, doctor, friend, parent*)

LIFE LESSON

....

Disrupted sleep patterns can cause your mental health to suffer so being able to create optimum conditions for sleep is essential. Understanding what is causing your sleep disruption is key to improving things.

TOPIC 10.7 I AM CONCERNED ABOUT MY ALCOHOL AND/OR DRUG INTAKE

Some people think drinking and drugs are an integral part of the university experience. However, you may feel uncomfortable using these substances if you do not like the way they make you feel, or they may be disallowed in your culture. Sometimes alcohol and drugs are seen as necessary for having a 'good time' and there can be a great deal of peer pressure involved to join in.

There are risks associated with both these substances, as well as the financial cost. Both are addictive meaning you may start to consume more over time, and they can also prevent conscious, logical thinking. This inability to think consciously does increase the chances of traumatic life events occurring such as drunken brawls, not being aware of date-rape drugs, unwanted pregnancies, accidents and even suicides. You may also be harming your body as there is a known link between drinking excessive alcohol, diabetes and cancer along with alcohol and drugs affecting neurological function long term. In addition, alcohol is a depressant and drugs can heighten symptoms of anxiety and paranoia.

You may think drinking alcohol means you have more fun, helps you relax, is a treat or even that you deserve it for working hard. You may feel more confident when you drink or have taken drugs. However, it is important to remember that you can have fun, relax, be sociable and confident without having to use these substances.

It is important to examine your behaviour in relation to alcohol and drugs. If you think you might be using alcohol or drugs to make a bad day better or to cheer yourself up, consider a more empowering and positive action to improve the way you feel. You might also drink alcohol and take drugs to fill an empty feeling inside, but it is better to try and fill this void by finding your purpose and passion in life.

Some young people use stimulants to make themselves feel better as they are unaware of alternative ways to feel good or have fun. However, society is slowly changing and more natural ways of getting high are becoming the norm. These include exercise, meditation, yoga, spending time in nature, finding one's true spiritual purpose, meaningful connections and exploring different spiritual healing modalities. Of course, these activities lead to increased feelings of purpose, improved physical and mental well-being, authentic connections and knowing you are part of something bigger than yourself. While chemical stimulants can make sometimes make you feel better in the short-term, these more spiritual activities lead to long-term happiness and improved mental health.

SELF-ENQUIRY REFLECTION 10.7

....

Being self-aware and honest about your behaviour in relation to alcohol and drugs and learning how to make conscious healthy choices is important in life. If you are using these substances to help mask other feelings and issues, you can learn to make healthier choices for your mental and physical well-being.

I have the courage to create healthier habits.

1. On a scale of 0–10 (10 being the maximum), how concerned am I about my alcohol and/or drug intake?

2. Where did I learn that alcohol and drugs are a way to feel better? (*Society, family, upbringing, friends, television, cultural norms*)

3. If I reduced my intake of these substances, how would this improve my life?

4. What would be my concerns about reducing my intake?

5. If I feel reliant on these substances, what action can I start to take to reduce this, and which other activities can I use to help heal myself?

LIFE LESSON

....

Letting go of a dependency on anything is important as it means it does not control you or have any power over you. Learning how to release attachment to or dependence on alcohol or drugs means YOU are in control of your life as you are not having to rely on these substances to make your reality better. You may need support in doing this and the resources section offers suggestions.

TOPIC 10.8 I THINK I HAVE AN ADDICTION AND I DON'T KNOW WHAT TO DO

The National Health Service defines addiction as 'not having control over doing, taking or using something to the point where it could be harmful to you'. It is extremely common for humans to be addicted to something through no fault of their own and it takes courage to admit you may have an addiction.

You may have become addicted to a substance, behaviour, way of thinking or even a person, as all these things can make you feel better in the short term. An addiction can make you feel happier, less sad, or even numb your feelings caused by what is happening around you – it can be seen as a self-soothing, sedating short-term activity helping you to get through a day. Alternatively, addictions hook you into feeling emotional highs and lows and this way of experiencing life may be all you know. This pattern of behaviour makes you feel in control, so you subconsciously choose behaviours or experiences which continue to make you feel this way.

However, the great news is you can heal from whatever addiction you think you have. If your current behaviour choices are causing you pain in some way, then recognising this is your point of change. You deserve to experience success, happiness, love and calmness in your life, and it is possible for you to achieve this. Once you learn to replace your addiction with healthy coping mechanisms you will feel much happier. Believing you have a right to be happy is your first step in changing your patterns of behaviour. You are lovable and deserve to be shown love both by yourself and others.

Please do not judge yourself for having an addiction of some sort. You have simply used a coping mechanism to help you survive each day which is understandable and brave. With the support and help of professionals, the universe and your own self will, you can discover the root cause as to why you are using unsuitable coping mechanisms to avoid facing your feelings and reality.

When you realise you are important and are a gift to the world, you will believe you do not need to self-sabotage your success by choosing to harm yourself through addictive behaviour. Healing any past pain you may have experienced is a spiritual journey worth taking, no matter how painful this journey may be at the time. There are many organisations that can help you, and many are listed in the resources section.

It is said that the most sensitive souls experience addictions as they struggle with how harsh some people can be on planet earth. Wanting to block out the cruelty they see, hear and feel is the only way they can cope. However, once you realise you have important gifts to help bring love and healing to the world, you can start to make more empowered choices in your life. The planet needs your wisdom right now.

SELF-ENQUIRY REFLECTION 10.8

. . . .

Realising you have an addiction can be your greatest gift as you start to heal the root cause of what has happened to you in your past which is making you want to change your reality. These questions will help you discern how you can take steps to get the help and support you need.

I have the courage to heal my addiction.

1. On a scale of 1–10 (10 being the maximum), how concerned am I that I may have an addiction to something or someone?

2. What do I think I am addicted to and why do I think this?

3. How does my reality change when I take the substance or partake in the addictive behaviour?

4. If I could heal my addiction, what benefits would this give me?

5. Who can I reach out to for support?
   (*Counsellor, tutor, friend, parent, doctor, support group, internet, higher power, energy healers, self-help books*)

LIFE LESSON

. . . .

Addictions are very common, especially in older people, therefore if you can heal your addiction now, it means you will increase the likelihood of living free from your addiction and the mental and emotional pain that comes with it. Seeking help is important to help you overcome your addiction.

TOPIC 10.9 | I HAVE HAD A BEREAVEMENT AND CAN'T STOP CRYING

....

A bereavement can be a life-altering and painful experience, especially at a young age. Bereavement brings loss and this is challenging due to the feelings that are triggered within such as anger, denial, grief or simply feeling numb. Grieving includes accepting all your feelings and not trying to escape them – important for your long-term mental health.

Grief can be an overwhelming emotion and it's important to allow yourself to cry when a memory is triggered, you have pangs of missing the person or you simply feel lonely. You may think crying is weak, however, this is untrue as crying is an act of bravery even though it can make you feel physically weak and out of control.

When grief becomes so bad you may think you don't want to be alive any-more it is important you do not judge or act on these thoughts and feelings and accept this is a completely understandable way to feel at this moment in time. However, please reach out to talk to someone who can help you.

It is also imperative that you try to resist numbing your feelings in any way with alcohol, food or drugs as these can stop you from processing and releas-ing your feelings. Not being afraid of feeling sad and upset is key to transitioning through your loss, helping you to reach a place of acceptance and peace.

You may feel relief if the person who has passed treated you cruelly and it is okay to feel this way. You may still grieve due to the betrayal and the loss of a relationship that you wanted but didn't get. It is important you do not judge your feelings as bad or feel guilty for feeling this way – how you feel is how you feel. Equally, you may not feel any emotions when someone close to you passes and this is okay too – it may just mean you didn't have a strong soul connection with them.

There is no time frame for grief so do not think you have to feel better within a week, month, a year or many years. However, if the loss is proving par-ticularly difficult to process you may find support in seeing a grief counsellor or someone who can help you explore how you feel. If you are comfortable with alternative therapies having some sort of energy healing or a session with a psychic medium may also help you.

SELF-ENQUIRY REFLECTION 10.9

....

You will experience losses throughout your life so understanding the emotional effects of bereavement is important. You may have lost a person, a pet, a stage in your life, a job, career, relationship or even a friendship. Processing your loss by feeling your emotions is an integral part of grieving. These questions will help you discern if you have truly grieved your losses.

I have the courage to feel my loss.

1. Who have I lost in my life and how do I feel when I think about this person?

If your bereavement was some time ago and yet you still come to tears when you think about this person or avoid thinking about this person, you may need support in helping you fully release the pain which still exists.

2. On a scale of 0–10 (10 being maximum), how much have I allowed myself to grieve (feel intense sorrow) or am allowing myself to grieve now?

3. How have I numbed my emotions or are numbing my emotions now?

4. How can I accept my feelings more and be okay sitting with my feelings?

5. How can I learn more about grieving the loss of someone or talk to someone who can help me?
   (*Internet, bereavement charity, counsellor, books, forums*)

LIFE LESSON

....

Being able to handle painful emotional life experiences is part of being human. Life is not about being happy all the time but being able to experience the full spectrum of your emotions as this gives your life meaning. If you have truly loved someone or something you will inevitably experience grief when they leave your life.

TOPIC 10.10 I HEAR VOICES IN MY HEAD AND DON'T KNOW WHAT TO DO

If voices in your head are telling you to harm yourself or another, then reach out for immediate support by phoning emergency services. The further reading and resources section at the back of this book offers sources of support.

Even though voice hearing is not common in the general population, please don't panic if you are currently experiencing this as not all voices in your head are damaging; in fact, some can be quite reassuring. The painful time is if your voice is telling you to do something which may harm you or another and this is the time when you must reach out for support.

You should visit your doctor who may direct you to a psychiatrist. You may also want to consider additional methods of support which can help you explore your past to discover why you are hearing voices.

Many who have recovered from hearing voices have done so from working in partnership with professionals who believe repressed pain from experiencing past trauma explains why you are hearing voices. They teach you ways to release this pain and therefore heal the voices. Accessing a more psychological healing programme may enable you to identify important messages to help you and this is why working with an alternative qualified practitioner can be beneficial.

The more psychologists investigate why people suffer with mental ill-health, the more they know to ask, 'What has happened in your past to make you feel this way?', rather than only asking 'What are you feeling right now?' This is because adverse childhood experiences and other factors are thought to predispose people to poor mental health. Gabor Mate, an author and physician, has conducted extensive research in this area and his books are listed in the resources section.

A more psycho-spiritual (non-religious) approach can support good mental health and being open to this way of healing may work for you. While there is always a place for the medical model, understanding that you are 'mind, body and spirit' is important for good mental health and living a happy, healthy and successful life. It is important you make an informed choice with your doctor or psychiatrist as to which type of treatment is right for you.

SELF-ENQUIRY REFLECTION 10.10

....

Being able to identify if your voices are helpful or sabotaging your happiness and success is important for your well-being. These questions will help you identify if you need to seek professional support (see resources section) or whether you are simply listening to your own thoughts which is quite normal.

I have the courage to reflect on the voice(s) in my head.

1. On a scale of 0–10 (10 being the maximum), how much am I hearing voice(s)?

2. What type of dialogue is being created by the voice(s)?
(*Helpful/unhelpful, safe/dangerous, narrator/dictator, loving/hateful*)

Many people have a voice in their head, it is simply a part of us narrating our day and while it may be negative, it is not destructive. However, if the voice feels like a dark force, telling you to harm yourself or another in any way then you need to access support now.

3. How are these voices affecting my daily life?

4. Who, of a more holistic nature can support me with these voices?

5. What research can you undertake to help you understand your past and why you may be hearing these voices now? (*See resource section*)

LIFE LESSON

....

Life can seem challenging sometimes but understanding where to access help for your mind, body and spirit is important. Being able to ask for help is a strength, not a weakness. The medical model will always be an option; however taking a holistic, spiritual approach is also worth considering.

TOPIC 10.11 I HAVE STARTED TO SELF-HARM, AND I DON'T WANT TO STOP

> If you feel like you want to self-harm now, put this book down and reach out to someone who is qualified to help you. This may be the emergency services or a professional trained to help you. You may think no one will understand how you are feeling but they will and may have even experienced it themselves. See the further reading and resources section at the back of this book for more support.

Self-harm is common, particularly in the 16–25 age group. You may have learned to harm yourself from a young age when you felt overwhelmed, scared, alone or unloved and so it is understandable you use this method to try and take your pain away. It may work in the short term to alleviate how you feel, however self-harming doesn't offer a long-term solution.

Common self-harm methods include:

- cutting body parts;
- banging or punching;
- scratching/pinching;
- hitting with objects;
- pulling hair out;

- ripping/tearing skin;
- punching walls and doors;
- carving into skin;
- burning skin;
- re-opening old wounds.

Whichever method you use, you may be self-harming to distract from, replace or remove the emotional pain you are feeling inside. This pain you are feeling may be 'historic pain'; if hurtful events occurred in your past and you didn't express the negative feelings of anger, rage, despair or hurt at the time then they are still within. These energies are wanting to be released and harming yourself can feel soothing in the short term. Think of a kettle when the water boils, the steam must be released from the spout – your body is no different and your feelings must be released to ensure you are mentally healthy. You may also be in a traumatic situation now and are using self-harm to cope with the overwhelming pain you currently feel.

Immediately after self-harming your current emotional pain may dissipate but unfortunately your historic pain is still there, meaning you may repeat the self-harming behaviour to experience the same feeling of relief. Therefore, self-harm can become an addiction, a coping mechanism to help you deal with uncomfortable feelings. You may also experience shame, sorrow and self-loathing after you have self-harmed which makes you feel worthless and unloved, so you are in a vicious circle. Show yourself love by acknowledging how brave you are to try and make yourself feel better but believe you can heal so you do not need to use this method in the future.

The depth of your current or historic pain and suffering is so deep that few people will understand why you self-harm; however, a professional will understand your struggle is real and that at the root is pain. Maybe something or someone in the past has caused you to think you are unimportant or unloved in some way? If someone or something has made you feel this way, this is not the truth and it is not your shame to carry any more, as the responsibility lay with them. Healing this core wound of shame will help you to think positively about yourself and realise you don't have to be your biggest bully, but that you are worthy of your own love, time and attention.

SELF-ENQUIRY REFLECTION 10.11

....

While self-harm can seem insurmountable, with the right awareness, support and intervention you can learn more positive coping mechanisms, meaning you live a life free from inflicting pain on yourself. You have a right to be happy and with the support of professionals, you can heal.

I have the courage to stop harming myself.

1. On a scale of 0–10, (10 being the maximum) how concerned am I about self-harming?

2. How do I feel *before, during* and *after* I have self-harmed?

3. What are my trigger points for self-harming?
   (*If you do not know, keep a diary of what happens and how it makes you feel before your self-harm*)

4. If I could find a more suitable way to manage how I feel, what would be the benefits of stopping self-harming?

5. As a first step towards healing, who can I talk to regarding self-harming? (*Self-help book, counsellor, lecturer, tutor, online groups, mentor, energy healer, doctor, friend*)

LIFE LESSON

....

During your life, you will have times of feeling emotionally overwhelmed and may use different coping mechanisms to help you feel better. Learning positive coping mechanisms means you can let go of unhelpful coping mechanisms and start to value the amazing, loving and worthy person you truly are.

TOPIC 10.12 I THINK I MAY HAVE AN EATING DISORDER

. . . .

The National Health Service in the UK defines an eating disorder as a 'condition where you use the control of food to cope with your feelings and other situations'. Unhealthy eating behaviours may include eating too much, too little and constantly worrying about your weight or body shape. You can recover from eating disorders, and it is important you find the right intervention for you.

One way to obtain support is via your doctor who may refer you to a specialist where you will be given support such as a controlled eating plan. This is not the only method of support and other interventions can be explored. What is important is you find the right plan for you.

Many people who have recovered from eating disorders felt as though there was a part of themselves which felt hopelessly unsatisfied and empty. This made them feel not good enough and anxious. Of course, the media and social media does not help by reinforcing that you should look a certain way in order to be accepted and loved. A wish to be thinner means you spend your time counting calories and may even be a way to keep some form of perceived control in your life.

As with other addictive behaviours, your eating disorder is often a way to manage distressing feelings, such as shame, anger and sadness, often derived from thinking you are unloved, unsafe or maybe because you once felt out of control and used food to make yourself feel better in some way. Even though your eating disorder may temporarily sedate this emotional distress, it does not remove uncomfortable feelings long term or change your thoughts regarding being unloved or unsafe.

Even if you arrived at university with your eating disorder, it is possible to leave university without it. Learning to accept all of your feelings and sit with how you feel is a true act of courage. This may be a painful place to be, but it is not as painful as carrying the physical, emotional and spiritual pain of your eating disorder.

Once you are ready to let go of your disorder, you will truly believe you are lovable, safe and here to make the world a better place: you can find an exciting new world filled with meaning, passion and purpose. Many people who have healed from an eating disorder go on to help others do the same. Reaching out for help by admitting your eating disorder is the first step to healthier eating habits and having a more positive body image.

SELF-ENQUIRY REFLECTION 10.12

....

An eating disorder can be a behaviour pattern which you perceive is helping you cope. Like any unhealthy habit, it can be unlearned and once you have found healthier ways to deal with your feelings, you will recover. These questions will help you discover how you can heal from your eating disorder

I have the courage to respect and nourish my body.

1. On a scale of 0–10 (10 being the maximum), how concerned am I about the eating disorder?

2. What is concerning me the most about the eating disorder?

3. How does the eating disorder benefit and sabotage me?
   (*It may benefit you by making you feel in control yet sabotage you as you cannot enjoy going out to a restaurant with your friends*)

4. What are my fears about obtaining help with the eating disorder?

5. What action can I take and where can I get help with my eating disorder?

LIFE LESSON

....

Finding positive ways to cope with your feelings is an essential part of maturation. You may be unsure how to release past or present emotional pain and it is understandable you have used food to feel better in some way. The important part is getting help so you do not continue to make yourself poorly. Your body is worthy of respect.

TOPIC 10.13 I FEEL SUICIDAL, AND I DON'T KNOW WHO TO ASK FOR HELP

I hope my words below will help if you are feeling this way, but as a first step remember there are people and organisations that you can reach out to immediately including the emergency services, **Nightline** and the **Samaritans**. See the further reading and resources section at the back of this book.

To not want to be alive anymore is possibly the worst feeling that you can experience. While the thought of ending your life may give you a solution from feeling the way you do, it also creates great despair. Your mind can be incessantly giving you horrendous negative messages such as, 'there is no point in being alive', 'I would be better off not here' and 'others would be happier without me in their life'. You may have even thought of ways to end your life and are planning how to do this currently. (Do be aware that certain substances such as alcohol and drugs can heighten suicidal thoughts.)

You may be wanting to end your life as you feel hopeless, you may be experiencing challenging life events such as a recent break-up, loss, or betrayal, or simply feel unloved and lonely. You may believe no one would care if you were not here anymore and therefore see no reason to stay. You may have lost all meaning to your life and your pain is so overwhelming you feel you want to go somewhere else which is not here.

However, let me reassure you that 'you are here on this planet for a reason'.

Scientists estimate the probability of you being born at about 1 in 400 trillion so please believe you are a *miracle*. The fact you were conceived means there is a reason for your existence – you simply have to find out what this reason is. You are meant to be here and have been created by the universe for a purpose. The American writer, Mark Twain said the two most important days in your life are the day you were born and the day you found out why. Perhaps it would help you to start to explore why you were born?

You may not want to talk to close friends or family for fear of upsetting them or because you don't think they will understand, but there are people and organisations who can offer you support at this most difficult of times and help you find out your raison d'être – reason for being (see the further reading section at the back of this book).

SELF-ENQUIRY REFLECTION 10.13

....

It is okay to feel how you feel at the moment, yet please be reassured that you can feel better with the right support. You may think ending your life is the best solution; however, it isn't. The most sensitive souls are often the ones who feel like they don't belong in this world, yet your sensitivity is what the world needs right now.

I have the courage to tell someone how I am really feeling.

1. On a scale of 0–10 (10 being the maximum), how much am I considering suicide?

The fact you are reading this book now and considering these questions indicates a wise, spiritual part of you knows suicide is not the answer. Listen more to this part of you.

2. On a scale of 0–10 (10 being the maximum) how much do I feel like I have a purpose in my life, a reason for being here?

If you have scored low on this question, this may explain why you do not want to be here. Please be reassured there is a purpose for you being here at the moment and you need to find out why.

3. Have you felt like this previously, and how did you find the courage to continue?

4. Who can you talk to right now about how you feel?
   (*Organisations like the Samaritans help people like you every day.*)

5. Where could you reach out to now?
   (*Please see the resources at the back of the book.*)

You may have experienced harshness and cruelty in your life growing up or you may be experiencing traumatic times right now. However, be reassured that there is someone out there who wants to help you remain here, realise how special you are and help you find your true purpose

LIFE LESSON

....

Not wanting to be alive is a feeling that you may experience from time to time in your life. You may feel it when life overwhelms you; however, if you know who to reach out for healing, support, love, and compassion, you will learn how to rebalance yourself so that you can feel better and back in control.

TOPIC 10.14 WHY DO I FEEL LOW AFTER I HAVE BEEN WITH SOME FAMILY OR FRIENDS?

Reflecting on how you feel after you have been in another's company is an important skill as being in another's company can affect your mental health. Their vibe may not resonate with yours anymore. You may have previously surrounded yourself with certain people but now you struggle to connect with them meaning you do not feel so inspired or happy after being with them.

It is important you find your tribe, which means:

- finding people who you enjoy being with and they enjoy being with you;
- you inspire each other to be a better person;
- you feel excited to see and listen to each other;
- having stimulating conversations and demonstrate respect for each other;
- finding those who open you up to new experiences and help you think in a more positive, empowering way.

Finding your tribe can improve your quality of life but also acknowledge that different friends do offer you different experiences. You may have one friend who is a really good listener but can be quite serious about life, another friend may not be such a good listener but is great fun to be with. Being able to have a tribe who together add to your life experience is a truly wonderful blessing indeed, however it is not the quantity of people in your tribe but the quality. Equally be aware of what you add to another's life experience – would someone want you as part of their tribe?

A key part of creating your tribe is knowing when to let go of those with whom you no longer resonate due to you evolving and changing as a person. Release any guilt of letting go of these people. Be mindful of having people in your life who bring you peace, solace and joy rather than simply because you share memories from the past.

You have the right to choose how you want to spend your valuable time. Spending time with people due to fear, obligation or guilt is not a positive place to be and will make you feel low and resentful. Being there for people who are in a low place in part may be an act of a good friend; however, taking care of yourself mentally and emotionally is being a good friend to yourself.

You may also be the type of person who enjoys their own company and does not need a lot of people around you. Embrace being a lone-wolf, as there is great solace in being alone. When the time is right, the universe will link you with your tribe, and equally you may be here to lead a new pack.

SELF-ENQUIRY REFLECTION 10.14

. . . .

Being able to reflect on how people add joy to your life and how you add joy to their life is a valuable use of your time. These questions will help you become aware of the type of people you want in your tribe and the type of person you want to be to others.

I have the courage to find my tribe.

1. How much on a scale of 0–10 (10 being the maximum), have I found my tribe?

2. Describe the type of people I would like in my tribe.

3. Describe the type of people I don't want in my tribe.

4. Describe the type of person I want to be in my tribe.

5. What action can I take to find my tribe, or am happy being a lone-wolf at the moment?

LIFE LESSON

. . . .

It is easy to stay connected with people simply because you have known them a long time as you may feel a loyalty to the times you shared and the memories you hold. However, if being with these people in the present day does not offer you the companionship that you seek then it may be time to let them go or seek new friends. As you evolve, the company you keep needs to evolve too.

TOPIC 10.15 HOW CAN SPIRITUALITY IMPROVE MY WELL-BEING?

You may not realise it, but you have a monologue in your head narrating a story from the time you awaken to the time you sleep. This is driven by your thoughts and these thoughts can be like an inner bully; critical, fear-based, full of shame and judgement, either about you as a person, others, or the world you live in. It is this narrative which can cause you emotional pain and contributes to poor mental health. Spirituality teaches you how to change this narrative into a more loving, encouraging and compassionate voice through a process called spiritual growth.

You are not born with this inner bully but may have learned it from your life experiences. You may have suffered criticism, judgement, harsh words or simply a lack of nurturing, validation and support in your past, either through society, people around you, your family, care-home or in your education. You may have been ignored, neglected, bullied or verbally punished and because of these experiences have a lack of love for yourself or distrust the universe.

Traversing the spiritual path teaches how to release any thoughts and feelings you hold such as '*I am unlovable, worthless or not enough*' and realise you are at your core consciousness of unconditional love. You realise you deserve to be loved and treated with respect and any unworthiness you feel is not your shame to carry. This shame originated in the person, people or society who influenced you growing up. Sadly, they probably did not feel good enough themselves, based on their upbringing, and may have repeated the cycle with you.

However, you can stop your shame from sabotaging you by realising you always were and are lovable, simply because you are a child of the universe. Your spiritual journey is to grow in self-belief and self-love, knowing you can handle challenging times, feel worthy of receiving good things and know there is a bigger plan for your life. Spiritual growth helps you increase your confidence by realising how powerful you are as a soul, helping you to transition difficult times of pain and suffering. As a result of walking your spiritual path, you have positive thoughts and feelings, meaning your mental health improves.

Spirituality also teaches of a divine intelligence in the universe, which is loving, guiding and able to create miracles. You cannot touch it or see it, but it is a knowing that you are being guided by a force bigger than yourself. You start to experience coincidences that your logical mind just cannot explain, and your feelings guide you to make empowering decisions. When you realise this divine intelligence is working for you, not against you, then you learn to let go and trust that you are guided and supported. Being spiritual is an inner journey of love for oneself and humanity and doesn't have to be connected to any religious doctrine or belief system.

SELF-ENQUIRY REFLECTION 10.15

Exploring your spiritual growth is an exciting journey as you learn to love the person you were born to be. These questions will help you if you are at the start of your spiritual journey, helping you to take the next steps in finding out more.

I have the courage to explore my spirituality.

1. On a scale of 0–10 (10 being the maximum), how aware am I of the negative narration in my head?

2. Where do I think I have developed this negative chatter from?
   (*Family, school, teachers, media, religion, friends, television, society*)

3. On a scale of 0–10 (10 being the maximum), how much do I feel I am lovable, and that I am supported by a divine intelligence?
   - *I am lovable =*
   - *I am supported by a divine intelligence =*

4. If I believed I was both of the above, how would this improve my mental health and day-to-day living?

5. Where can I start to explore my spirituality?
   (*Internet, books, friends, groups, social media, meditation, apps, spiritual therapists*)

LIFE LESSON

Being spiritual is not the same as being religious as you do not follow a set of external rules, beliefs or doctrines. Being spiritual is an inner journey of learning to love and respect yourself. The resources section offers further sources of spiritual support.

CONCLUSION

I would like to conclude *You've Got This* by sharing a piece of writing which I repeat when I am feeling angry, confused, helpless, sad or even just overcome by fear. I came across it after attending a weekly 12-step group called Al-Anon. Here I shared time with kind souls who offered me understanding and compassion while I traversed an emotionally challenging time. After completing the 12-step programme (thank you Wanda) which the group advocates, I learned the true power of surrendering to divine intelligence.

At the end of each meeting, we closed with the serenity prayer and were encouraged to repeat it throughout the week when experiencing emotional discomfort.

> *God,* grant me the Serenity*
> *To accept the things I cannot change*
> *Courage to change the things I can,*
> *And Wisdom to know the difference.*

*Like me, you may be uncomfortable using the word God so please replace it with a word which suits your beliefs.

I share this with you now as throughout your university life and beyond you will have many different experiences, some good and some which, through no fault of your own, will be painful and unable to be changed. Therefore, find the soul lesson in the experience and trust in your ability to handle it. Please believe the tough times will pass, as they always do.

You will also have times where you realise you are in emotional pain but need to find the courage to take action to change the situation,

CONCLUSION

allowing you to walk away from the pain. While this too can also be emotionally turbulent, your confidence will increase as you realise you can use your personal power to shift from a place of emotional turmoil to one of peace.

Knowing the difference between what you can and can't change is called wisdom and is learned through experience. I trust this book has given you suggestions to practice exerting your personal power to change challenging situations, thus allowing you to feel at peace.

May you find this mantra as beneficial I have.

From one brave soul to another

Rachael
rachael-alexander.com

FURTHER READING AND SOURCES OF SUPPORT

There are many different people who can support you while you are at university, from accommodation officers to the careers service. For more personal support, you can contact your personal tutor who may also be called, personal academic tutor, academic support tutor, academic tutor, or academic mentor. There is no need to suffer in silence and you are not alone.

There are also many external sources of support which you can access. The following are suggestions but not an exhaustive list. I can personally recommend many of them as they have been helpful on my own personal and spiritual journey.

HELP WITH PERSONAL AND SPIRITUAL GROWTH

Bradshaw, J (1991) *Homecoming – Reclaiming and Championing Your Inner Child*. London: Little Brown Book Group.

Carnes, P. J. & Phillips, B (2019) *The Betrayal Bond Breaking Free of Exploitive Relationships*. Florida: Health Communications Inc.

Cooper, D (1998) *The Power of Inner-Peace*. London: Piatkus.

Engel, B (2006) *Healing Your Emotional Self – A Powerful Program to Help You Raise Your Self-Esteem, Quiet Your Inner-Critic and Overcome Your Shame*. London: John Wiley & Sons.

FURTHER READING AND SOURCES OF SUPPORT

Gibson, L. C (2015) *Adult Children of Emotionally Immature Parents – How to Heal From Distant, Rejecting, or Self-Involved Parents.* Oakland: New Harbinger Publications.

Hay, L (1984) *You can heal your life.* London: Hay House.

Hay, L (1990) *Love yourself, heal your life workbook.* London: Hay House.

Jeffers, S (2007) *Feel the Fear and Do It Anyway®.* (revised edition). London: Vermillion.

King, V (2021) *Healing Is the New High: A Guide to Overcoming Emotional Turmoil and Finding Freedom.* London: HayHouse UK.

Miller, A (2008) *The Drama of Being a Child – The Search for your True Self.* London: Little Brown Book Group.

Orloff, J (2017) *The Empaths Survival Guide – Life Strategies for Sensitive People.* Canada: Sounds True.

Redfield, J (1984) *The Celestine Prophecy: How to Refresh Your Approach to Tomorrow with a New Understanding, Energy and Optimism.* London: Bantam.

Roman, S (1988) *Spiritual Growth – Being Your Higher Self (Earth Life)2.* Ohio: Kramer.

Ruiz, D. M (2017) *The Mastery of Self: A Toltec Guide to Personal Freedom.* Texas: Heirophant.

Singer, M. A (2007) *The Untethered Soul - The Journey Beyond Yourself.* Oakland: Harbinger.

Tolle, E (2009) *A New Earth – Awakening to your Life's Purpose.* London: Viking Books.

Vale, J (2011) *Kick the Drink… Easily.* London: CrownHouse.

Wauters, A (1996) *Journey of Self Discovery. How to work with the energies of Chakras and Archetypes.* London: Piatkus.

Williamson, M (1996) *A Return to Love. Reflections on The Principles of A Course in Miracles.* London: HarperCollins.

UNDERSTANDING PSYCHIATRIC DIAGNOSES, DRUGS USED AND WHY YOU MAY FEEL THE WAY YOU DO

Davies, J (2013) *Cracked - Why Psychiatry is Doing More than Harm Than Good*. London: Ikon.

Hari, J (2018) *Lost Connections Why You're Feeling Depressed and How to Find Hope*. London: Bloomsbury.

Kirsch, I (2009) *The Emperor's New Drugs – Exploding the Antidepressant Myth*. London: Random House.

Johnstone, L (2014) *A Straight Talking Introduction to Psychiatric Diagnosis*. Monmouth: PCCS Books.

Moncrieff, J (2009) *A Straight Talking Introduction to Psychiatric Drugs*. Monmouth: PCCS Books.

Mate, G (2018) *In The Realm of Hungry Ghosts – Close encounters with Addiction*. London: Penguin Random House.

Mate, G (2019) *When The Body Says No – The Cost of Hidden Stress*. London: Penguin Random House.

Van Der Kolk, B (2015) *The Body Keeps The Score – Mind, Body and Brain in The Transformation of Trauma*. London: Penguin Random House.

PSYCHOLOGICAL AND SPIRITUAL HEALING MODALITIES

You may like to explore the following. Try to use recommendations where possible and use your intuition as to whether the person appears kind, honest, trustworthy and displays integrity.

- akashic records
- angelic healing
- astrology (I recommend suedibnah.com)
- Bach flower remedies
- coaching
- Centre for Excellence Online Training Courses

- colour healing
- counselling
- crystal healing
- emotional freedom technique
- gong bath healing
- inner-child healing
- journaling
- kinesiology (I recommend philclubley.co.uk)
- massage
- mindfulness (I recommend the Insight Timer app)
- meditation and visualisation (I recommend glennharrold.com)
- oracle cards
- psychic/mediumship (I recommend suwalker.co.uk)
- reflexology
- reiki healing
- shaman healing
- solfeggio frequency healing
- soul retrieval (I recommend suegrassby.com)
- vibrational healing
- yoga

HELPFUL ORGANISATIONS
....

- 12 step-groups
- Beat Eating Disorders
- hearing-voices.org
- MIND
- NSPA.Org (suicide prevention)
- Samaritans
- SANE

USEFUL PSYCHOLOGICAL THEORIES

- Assertiveness including the *Assertive Bill of Rights*
- Attachment theory
- Co-dependency
- Karpman Drama Triangle
- Inner-child work
- Transactional analysis
- Trauma bonding

ORGANISATIONS* THAT WORK DIRECTLY TO SUPPORT STUDENTS WITH THEIR MENTAL HEALTH

••

- Charlie Waller Trust
- Nightline
- Papyrus
- Students Against Depression
- Student Minds
- Students Union

ORGANISATIONS THAT INDIRECTLY SUPPORT STUDENTS WITH THEIR MENTAL HEALTH

••

- Alliance for Student Led Wellbeing
- AMOSSHE
- Mental Wellbeing in Higher Education
- Smarten
- Student Health Association
- University Mental Health Advisory Network

Apologies to any support groups omitted, please contact the publisher if you would like to be consider for inclusion in further reprints

INDEX

INDEX

INDEX

INDEX